Acute Pain Management

A Practical Guide

Commissioning Editor: Serena Bureau
Project Development Manager: Francesca Lumkin
Project Manager: Hilary Hewitt
Project Controller: Mark Sanderson
Designer: Ian Dick

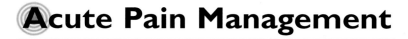

Acute Pain Management

A Practical Guide

SECOND EDITION

PAMELA E MACINTYRE BMEDSC, MBBS, MHA, FANZCA, FFPMANZCA
Director, Acute Pain Service
Department of Anaesthesia and Intensive Care
Royal Adelaide Hospital and University of Adelaide
Adelaide, Australia

L BRIAN READY MD, FRCP(C)
Professor, Department of Anesthesiology
Director, UWMC Pain Service
University of Washington
Seattle, USA

W.B. Saunders

London · Edinburgh · New York · Philadelphia · St Louis · Sydney · Toronto · 2001

W.B. SAUNDERS
An imprint of Elsevier Science Limited

First edition published in 1996
Reprinted 2002

ISBN 07020 2581X

British Library Cataloguing in Publication Data
A catalogue record for this book is available from the British Library

Library of Congress Cataloging in Publication Data
A catalog record for this book is available from the Library of
Congress

Note
Medical knowledge is constantly changing. As new information
becomes available, changes in treatment, procedures, equipment and
the use of drugs become necessary. The authors and the publishers
have taken care to ensure that the information given in this text is
accurate and up to date. However, readers are strongly advised to
confirm that the information, especially with regard to drug usage,
complies with the latest legislation and standards of practice.

The
publisher's
policy is to use
**paper manufactured
from sustainable forests**

Typeset by IMH(Cartrif), Loanhead, Scotland
Printed in China

CONTENTS

O ver the past few years, increasing emphasis has been placed on the need to improve the management of acute pain. As well as increasing patient comfort, better pain relief may also improve outcome after surgery or injury in some patients.

The first edition of this book aimed to provide nurses, medical students and doctors in training (interns, house officers, residents and registrars) with simple and practical information and guidelines that would help them to better manage their patients' pain. It was intended to give a better understanding of the conventional methods of analgesia as well as the newer techniques available for the treatment of acute pain, such as patient-controlled and epidural analgesia. It was also hoped that the book would be of some use to other general and specialist medical practitioners with an interest in the treatment of acute pain; especially those who were introducing changes to the way acute pain was managed in their institution.

Since the first edition, newer drugs have become available for use in acute pain management and there have been some changes in the techniques used. Importantly, there has also been increasing recognition of the need to individualize treatment in order to obtain the best results for each patient.

In the second edition of this book, all chapters have been updated and new drugs and techniques included. In addition, new chapters have been added to assist in the management of three groups of patients in whom acute pain management can be a little more challenging – opioid-dependent patients, patients with acute neuropathic pain, and elderly patients. A self-assessment section at the end has also been added, with examples of questions that may form part of a hospital acute pain management accreditation program.

We are grateful to our anesthesiology and nursing colleagues for their comments and suggestions for both editions and in particular to Acute Pain Service nurses Judith, Kevin and Leesa for reviewing the drafts of the new edition.

The second edition remains a practical book only and detailed information about the anatomy, neurochemistry and pathophysiology of acute pain has been omitted. It is not possible for a book of this size to contain detailed information on every drug and every technique used for the management of acute pain. Suggested drugs, doses and treatment regimens are guidelines only and may have to be adapted according to different patients and clinical situations.

Pamela E. Macintyre
L. Brian Ready
2000

CHAPTER 1

INTRODUCTION

Why should acute pain management be improved?

Results of better acute pain management

Acute pain services

Measurement of pain

Since the 1960s, studies of adult hospital patients have consistently highlighted inadequacies in the treatment of acute pain, with over 80% of patients in some surveys reporting moderate to severe pain in the postoperative period. Patients with other causes of acute pain, such as burns, multiple trauma, or illnesses such as pancreatitis or myocardial infarction, have fared no better. Some of the reasons often cited for poor analgesia are:

- a belief that pain is not harmful to the patient or that it is a 'normal' consequence of surgery and injury
- concerns that pain relief will obscure a surgical diagnosis or mask the signs of surgical complications
- a tendency to underestimate a patient's pain and not recognize the variability in patients' perceptions of pain
- lack of regular and frequent assessment of pain and any pain-relieving measures
- fears that the patient will become addicted to opioids
- concerns of a high risk of respiratory depression with opioids
- inadequate preoperative patient education regarding postoperative analgesia
- patient reluctance to request analgesia
- lack of understanding of the enormous interpatient variability in opioid requirements
- lack of recognition that age is a better predictor of opioid requirement than weight in the adult patient

1

- prolonged dosing intervals and a belief that opioids must not be given more often than every 4 hours
- insufficient flexibility in dosing schedules (dose and dose intervals)
- lack of understanding of the need to titrate analgesics to meet the needs of each patient
- lack of accountability for pain management

In the 1990s, increasing emphasis was placed on the need for better acute pain management, with the aims of improving patient comfort and outcome after surgery. A number of major bodies worldwide, recognizing this need, published recommendations and guidelines for the treatment of acute pain. These include:

- Royal College of Surgeons and College of Anaesthetists (1990): *Report of the Working Party on Pain after Surgery*
- Faculty of Anaesthetists and Royal Australasian College of Surgeons (1991): *Statement on Acute Pain Management*
- International Association for the Study of Pain, Task Force on Acute Pain (Ready and Edwards, 1992): *Management of Acute Pain: A Practical Guide*
- US Department of Health and Human Services, Agency for Health Care Policy and Research (1992): *Clinical Practice Guideline for Acute Pain Management*
- American Society of Anesthesiologists (Ready et al., 1995): *Practice Guidelines for Acute Pain Management in the Perioperative Setting*
- National Health and Medical Research Council, Australia (1999): *Acute Pain Management: The Scientific Evidence*

These reports and guidelines stress that a patient has the right to expect adequate treatment of acute pain and that all members of the health care team have an ethical obligation to provide it. The ethical importance is further increased when additional benefits, such as improved outcome, are considered.

Recent improvements in acute pain management have been due largely to the introduction of new techniques for the delivery of analgesic drugs (e.g. patient-controlled and epidural analgesia), a growing interest in this area among anesthesiologists, and the establishment of acute pain services (see later).

However, despite these advances and despite the reports above, pain management remains unsatisfactory for many patients. Studies from the mid to late 1990s suggest that up to three-quarters of postoperative patients are still reporting moderate to severe pain.

Pain relief for patients prescribed one of the more traditional analgesic techniques (e.g. intermittent intramuscular opioid analgesia) commonly remains inadequate. Even newer methods of pain relief are not always successful. For example, patient-controlled analgesia (PCA) can provide excellent and safe pain relief if conditions exist that facilitate its effective use. However, if a patient is just given a PCA machine, with inadequately trained nursing and medical staff and without adequate explanation of the technique, results may be disappointing, if not hazardous. On the other hand, with adequate training of staff, involvement of the patient, and the use of more flexible dosing regimens, even simple injections of morphine can be effective.

Improvements in acute pain management must aim at better analgesia for all patients. More important than the individual drug or analgesic technique is the need to learn the principles of *individual* pain control and the ability to recognize and address the various barriers to effective pain relief listed above. Education of patients, medical students, nursing students and staff (see Chapter 12), and the provision of guidelines for simple as well as advanced methods of analgesia, therefore play an important role. Regular and routine assessments of pain and any side effects of pain relief should be performed and documented just as a patient's other 'vital signs' – blood pressure, pulse, respiratory rate and temperature – are recorded on a regular basis. This will serve to make pain 'visible' and allow better titration of analgesia for each patient.

WHY SHOULD ACUTE PAIN MANAGEMENT BE IMPROVED?

In the past, many medical and nursing personnel believed that pain was a natural, inevitable, acceptable and harmless consequence of surgery and trauma. However, pain and postoperative nausea and vomiting are the major preoperative concerns of many patients. It is also recognized that undertreatment of severe acute pain, coupled with the physiological response to surgery known as the stress response, can have a number of adverse consequences – see **Box 1.1**.

CARDIOVASCULAR SYSTEM

Severe pain increases sympathetic nervous system activity and levels of circulating catecholamines, resulting in rises in heart rate, blood pressure and peripheral vascular resistance. These in turn increase the workload of the heart and the oxygen consumption of the myocardium. Myocardial oxygen supply may already be decreased owing to cardiac or respiratory disease or as a result of hypoxemia from the postoperative pulmonary changes

Possible harmful effects of undertreated severe acute pain

Cardiovascular	Tachycardia, hypertension, increased peripheral vascular resistance, increased myocardial oxygen consumption, myocardial ischemia, altered regional blood flow, deep vein thrombosis	
Respiratory	Decreased lung volumes, atelectasis, decreased cough, sputum retention, infection, hypoxemia	
Gastrointestinal	Decreased gastric and bowel motility	
Genitourinary	Urinary retention	
Neuroendocrine/ metabolic	Increased catabolic hormones:	catecholamines, cortisol, glucagon, growth hormone, vasopressin, aldosterone, renin and angiotensin
	Reduced anabolic hormones:	insulin, testosterone
Musculoskeletal	Muscle spasm, immobility (increasing risk of deep vein thrombosis)	
Psychological	Anxiety, fear, sleeplessness	
Chronic pain		

Box 1.1

outlined below. If oxygen consumption is greater than oxygen supply, myocardial ischemia (which may be silent in the postoperative period) will result.

Increased sympathetic stimulation may also alter regional blood flow, directing blood away from skin and viscera towards brain and heart. Decreased blood flow may impair wound healing and increase muscle spasm.

Severe pain may reduce patient mobility and promote venous stasis. Increases in fibrinogen and platelet activation will increase blood coagulability. Both of these factors will increase the risk of deep vein thrombosis and pulmonary embolism.

RESPIRATORY SYSTEM

Pain from operation or injury to the chest or abdomen can exaggerate pulmonary dysfunction, resulting in splinting of the muscles of the diaphragm and chest wall and an impaired ability to cough. This leads to a reduction in lung volumes (vital capacity, forced expiratory volume and functional residual capacity), atelectasis and sputum retention, which can result in hypoxemia and an increased risk of chest infections. Postoperative pulmonary changes are most pronounced on the first or second day after surgery and may take 2 weeks or more to return to preoperative values.

GASTROINTESTINAL AND GENITOURINARY SYSTEMS

Pain can lead to significant delays in gastric emptying and a reduction in intestinal motility. This is thought to be mainly due to activation of a spinal reflex arc. Other causes of inhibition of motility in the postoperative period include opioid administration and surgery. After abdominal surgery, colonic motility is inhibited for 48–72 hours, while motility in the stomach and small intestine usually recovers within 12–24 hours. Urinary retention may also occur.

NEUROENDOCRINE AND METABOLIC SYSTEMS

Pain is believed to play a major part in the activation of the neuroendocrine 'stress response' seen after surgery or trauma and resulting in the release of a number of hormones (see **Box 1.1**).

These changes can lead to hyperglycemia, increases in fibrinogen and platelet activation (increased coagulability), increased protein breakdown and a negative nitrogen balance, and impairments of wound healing and immune function (with a consequent decreased resistance to infection). Sodium and water retention may also occur. The increase in metabolic rate will further increase demands on the cardiorespiratory system.

MUSCULOSKELETAL SYSTEM
Muscle spasm may reduce respiratory function, and immobility will increase the possibility of venous stasis and deep vein thrombosis.

PSYCHOLOGICAL EFFECTS
Untreated pain can lead to, or increase, patient anxiety, fear, sleeplessness and fatigue. Aggressive or belligerent behaviour may be a sign of anxiety and distress.

CHRONIC PAIN
Occasionally patients develop chronic pain after surgery or other injury. While some may have suffered some form of nerve damage (see Chapter 10), the cause in others remains unexplained. It is possible that the risk of development of chronic pain is higher in those patients with severe acute pain.

RESULTS OF BETTER ACUTE PAIN MANAGEMENT

Effective analgesia can at least partially reverse some of the harmful effects outlined above and will assist in early mobilization and rehabilitation of the patient. Thus, treatment of acute pain is important not only for the humanitarian reasons of patient comfort and satisfaction, but also because it may significantly improve outcome by reducing the incidence of postoperative complications and shortening hospital stay, especially in the high-risk patient. Epidural analgesia, for example, has been shown to decrease the risk of pulmonary and cardiac complications in the postoperative period and to allow earlier return of bowel function.

To gain the maximum benefit from pain relief, effective analgesia must be accompanied by effective postoperative rehabilitation regimens.

PRE-EMPTIVE ANALGESIA

Pre-emptive analgesia is pain-relieving therapy given to patients prior to the onset of pain. The aim is to prevent changes in the spinal cord that occur with repetitive input of painful stimuli from the site of injury, and which may lead to an exaggerated response to pain, in terms of both magnitude and duration.

The benefits of pre-emptive analgesia have been shown in animal studies. It had been hoped that similar advantages would be seen in surgical patients and that this would lead to less pain in the immediate postoperative period and in the longer term. However, clinical studies have been disappointing. In part this may reflect the fact that pain after surgery and injury results from extensive tissue damage leading to ongoing painful stimuli, whereas such damage in experimental studies may be more restricted. The benefits of pre-emptive analgesia are more likely to be seen if an effective block of these painful stimuli is achieved and if analgesia is continued over the entire duration of the high-intensity stimuli.

While evidence of any clinical advantage in the short term is still inconsistent, there are some data to suggest that long-term benefits may occur. Some studies, using pre-emptive analgesia and aggressive approaches to the management of postoperative pain, have been able to show a reduction in the incidence of subsequent chronic pain. Some of these studies have focused on pain after limb amputation, and have been able to show that the incidence of phantom pain is significantly less when epidural analgesia is commenced preoperatively and continued into the postoperative period.

ACUTE PAIN SERVICES

The first anesthesiologist-based acute pain service (APS) in the USA was started by Ready in 1986. Since that time many

7

hospitals worldwide have followed suit and the number continues to grow. Common to the reports listed earlier is the recommendation that all major acute care centers should establish acute pain teams or services.

There has been some debate as to the best form of acute pain service. Suggested models fall into two main groups: physician-based (usually run by anesthesiologists because the knowledge required and techniques used are similar to those used in anesthesia) and nurse-based. Regardless of the model chosen, an organized team approach is important.

The nurse-based, anesthesiologist-supervised model described by Rawal and Berggren (1994) seeks to involve all nurses in the provision of better analgesia, regardless of technique used. They propose that improved education and regular monitoring of pain and pain relief ('making pain visible') will lead to better analgesia for all patients. There are also significant advantages in terms of cost. It has been shown that the appointment of an acute pain nurse to a hospital can improve the effectiveness of all forms of pain relief.

Unfortunately, some anesthesiologist-based acute pain services have tended to concentrate on the 'high-tech' approaches to pain relief and placed much less emphasis on improving the simple methods of pain relief throughout their hospital. This approach benefits only a small proportion of patients. This need not be the case, as the organization of an APS can be such that pain management for all patients in the institution will improve. As with the nurse-based service, an anesthesiologist-based APS should assist in the development of undergraduate and postgraduate education programs and better protocols for all analgesic techniques used throughout the hospital (**Box 1.2**).

Anesthesiologist-based services may also have other advantages. The APS anesthesiologists will have expert knowledge about the pharmacology of all analgesic agents, the different delivery techniques available, and the risks and benefits of these techniques. They may therefore be more likely to tailor 'standard' orders to suit individual patients. They will also have a good understanding of the disease processes of the patients they are seeing, and may be called on to help with acute postoperative

Role of an acute pain service

1. *Education (initial, updates)*
   anesthesiologists
   surgeons
   junior medical staff
   pharmacists
   hospital administrators
   nurses (accreditation/reaccreditation programs)
   patients and families
   medical and nursing students
   physiotherapists
   health insurance carriers
2. *Introduction and supervision of more advanced analgesic techniques including:*
   patient-controlled analgesia
   epidural and intrathecal analgesia
   other continuous regional analgesia techniques
3. *Assistance in improving traditional analgesic treatment regimens including:*
   intermittent opioid regimens (IM, SC, IV and oral)
4. *Standardization of:*
   equipment
   'standard orders' for advanced analgesic techniques
   • drugs, doses and drug dilutions
   • diagnosis and treatment of side effects
   • specific monitoring requirements for each analgesic technique
   nursing procedure protocols
   guidelines for the monitoring of all patients receiving opioids
   guidelines for the use of other analgesic drugs and adjuvant agents
   nondrug treatment orders, e.g. use of oxygen, use of antireflux valves
5. *24-hour availability of pain service personnel*
   for advice about any pain management problems as well as for
   patients under the care of the APS
6. *Collaboration and communication with other medical and nursing services including:*
   chronic pain clinics
   drug and alcohol services
   surgical services
7. *Regular audit of activity and continuous quality improvement*
8. *Clinical research*

Box 1.2

problems. When 'high-tech' options such as PCA are used, patients whose pain relief is managed by an anesthesiologist-based APS may have less pain, suffer fewer side effects and express greater satisfaction, than patients whose PCA is supervised by less experienced medical staff.

MEASUREMENT OF PAIN

The International Association for the Study of Pain (IASP) defines pain as '*An unpleasant sensory and emotional experience associated with actual or potential tissue damage or described in terms of such damage*' (IASP, 1979).

Pain is a very individual experience and there are a host of behavioral, psychological and social factors that may increase or decrease the patient's response to, and report of, pain. These factors may include previous pain experiences, cultural background, social supports, the meaning and consequences of the pain (e.g. disease or surgical prognosis, loss of employment), coping styles, degree of control felt over the pain and disease, and fear, anxiety or depression. These will interact to produce what the patient then describes as pain. Not surprisingly, there is often a poor correlation between the patient's assessment of pain and the nursing or medical staff's estimate of the pain that the patient is experiencing.

There are a number of simple clinical techniques available for assessment and measurement of pain and its response to treatment. The best methods involve self-reporting by the patient rather than observer assessment. Observation of behavior and/or vital signs is an unreliable measure of pain and should not be used alone unless the patient is unable to communicate. Discrepancies between patients' behavior and their self-report of pain may result from differences in the factors listed above, which can modulate the amount of pain experienced.

If a patient is unable to give a self-report of pain, functional assessment may be less biased than observation of behavior and vital signs. The ability to take deep breaths, cough, ambulate and cooperate with physiotherapy may give some indication of the effectiveness of analgesic therapy.

In adults, three common methods of pain measurement using patient self-report are the visual analog scale, the verbal numerical rating scale and the categorical rating scale. Each of these methods is reasonably reliable as long as any endpoints and adjectives employed are carefully selected and standardized. While often used to compare levels of pain between patients, these methods of scoring pain are probably of most use as measures of change in the level of pain within each patient and the effectiveness of treatment of that pain. Studies show a good correlation between these measures of pain.

COMMONLY USED MEASURES OF PAIN
Visual analog scale

The visual analog scale (VAS) uses a 10 cm line with endpoint descriptors such as 'no pain' marked at the left end of the line and 'worst pain imaginable' marked at the right end. There are no other cues marked on the line. The patient is asked to mark a point on the line that best represents the pain. The distance from 'no pain' to the patient's mark is then measured and this equals the VAS score.

No pain   Worst pain imaginable

To simplify these measurements, VAS slide rules have been developed. On the front of the slide rule is a 10 cm line with the endpoints such as 'no pain' and 'worst pain imaginable'. The reverse side of the slide rule shows the same line marked at millimeter intervals. The patient moves the slide along the line on the front of the slide rule to the point that best represents the pain. The corresponding VAS measurement is then read off the back of the slide rule.

The disadvantages of the VAS system are that it can be more time-consuming than other simple scoring methods, specific equipment is needed (albeit very simple equipment), and some patients may have difficulty understanding or performing this score, especially in the immediate postoperative period. One advantage of this method is that the wording can be written in many different languages.

The VAS scale can also be adapted to measure other variables such as patient satisfaction, pain relief and nausea.

Verbal numerical rating scale

The verbal numerical rating scale (VNRS) is similar to the VAS. Patients are asked to imagine that '0 equals no pain' and '10 equals the worst pain imaginable' and then to give a number on this scale that would best represent the pain. The advantage of this type of system is that it does not require any equipment. However, problems may occur if there is a language barrier or the patient has some other difficulty in understanding the scoring system.

Verbal descriptor scale

The verbal descriptor scale (VDS) uses different words to rate pain, such as *none, mild, moderate, severe.*

WHAT PAIN SCORE IS 'COMFORTABLE'?

It is usually not possible, practical or safe to aim for complete pain relief at all times with most of the drugs and drug administration techniques currently used in the treatment of acute pain. The aim of treatment should be patient comfort, both at rest and with physical activity such as coughing or ambulation.

 Just as pain is a very individual experience, the correlation of 'comfort' and a specific pain score may show marked interpatient variability. Therefore, alterations in analgesic regimens may need to take into account a number of factors such as the patients' pain score, the level that they would regard as comfortable, and their functional ability, e.g. ability to take deep breaths, cough or walk. The presence or absence of any side effects from analgesic drugs will also affect what alterations are made to treatment orders. Alterations based solely on a particular pain score may lead to excessive treatment in some patients, and undertreatment in others.

High pain scores may not always require the dose of an analgesic to be increased. This does not mean that the patient's report of pain is disbelieved, but that the appropriate therapeutic response to the reported pain may vary between individual patients. For example, patients who are very anxious may report high pain levels, yet treatment (not necessarily drug treatment) of that anxiety, rather than an automatic increase in analgesic dose, may be preferable. Other patients may have pain which is not always responsive to opioid drugs and which may require treatment using other classes of analgesic drugs (e.g. neuropathic pain – See Chapter 10).

WHEN SHOULD PAIN BE MEASURED?

Patients are usually asked to rate their pain when they are resting. However, a better indicator of the effectiveness of analgesia is an assessment of the pain caused by physical activity such as coughing, deep breathing or movement. Therefore, pain scores at rest and with movement or coughing should be recorded.

Pain should be reassessed regularly during the postoperative period. The frequency of assessment should be increased if the pain is poorly controlled or if the pain stimulus or treatment interventions are changing.

REFERENCES AND FURTHER READING

Bach S., Noreng M.F. and Tjellden N.U. (1988) Phantom limb in amputees during the first 12 months following limb amputation after preoperative lumbar epidural blockade. *Pain* 33, 297–310.

Ballantyne J.C., Carr D.B., Chalmers T.C. et al. (1993) Postoperative patient-controlled analgesia: meta-analyses of initial randomised control trials. *Journal of Clinical Anesthesia* 5, 182–193.

Ballantyne J.C., Carr D.B., deFerranti S. et al. (1998) The comparative effects of postoperative analgesic therapies on pulmonary outcome: cumulative meta-analyses of randomized, controlled trials. *Anesthesia and Analgesia* 86, 598–612.

Carr D.B., Jacox A.K., Chapman R.C. et al. (1992) *Acute Pain Management: Operative or Medical Procedures and Trauma, Clinical Practice Guideline.* AHCPR Pub. No. 92-0032. Rockville, MD: Agency for Health Care Policy and Research, Public Health Service, US Department of Health and Human Services.

Coleman S.A. and Booker-Milburn J. (1996) Audit of postoperative pain control: influence of a dedicated acute pain nurse. *Anaesthesia* 51, 1093–1096.

Collins S.L., Moore R.A. and McQuay H.J. (1997) The visual analogue pain intensity scale: what is moderate pain in millimetres? *Pain* 72, 95–97.

Dahl J.B. (1995) The status of pre-emptive analgesia. *Current Opinion in Anaesthesiology* 8, 323–330

Faculty of Anaesthetists and Royal Australasian College of Surgeons (1991) *Statement on Acute Pain Management.* Melbourne.

Gould T.H., Crosby D.L., Harmer M. et al. (1992) Policy for managing pain control after surgery: effect of sequential changes in management. *British Medical Journal* 305, 1187–1193.

Harmer M. and Davies K.A. (1998) The effect of education, assessment and a standardised prescription on postoperative pain management. *Anaesthesia* **53**, 424–430.

IASP Subcommittee on Taxonomy (1979) Pain terms: a list with definitions and notes on usage. *Pain* **6**, 249–252.

Liu S., Carpenter R.L. and Neal J.M. (1995) Epidural anesthesia and analgesia: their role in postoperative outcome. *Anesthesiology* **82**, 1474–1506.

Macintyre P.E., Runciman W.B.R. and Webb R.K. (1990) An acute pain service in an Australian teaching hospital – the first year. *Medical Journal of Australia* **153**, 417–420.

Meissner A., Rolf N. and Van Aken H. (1997) Thoracic epidural anesthesia and the patient with heart disease: risks and controversies. *Anesthesia and Analgesia* **85**, 517–528.

Miaskowski C., Crews J., Ready L.B. et al. (1999) Anesthesia-based pain services improve the quality of postoperative pain management. *Pain* **80**, 23–29.

National Health and Medical Research Council (1999) *Acute Pain Management: The Scientific Evidence.* Canberra (available at http://www.nhmrc.health.gov.au/publicat/pdf/cp57.pdf)

Rawal N. and Berggren L. (1994) Organization of acute pain service: a low cost model. *Pain* **57**, 117–123.

Ready L.B. and Edwards W.T. (eds) (1992) *Management of Acute Pain: A Practical Guide.* IASP Task Force on Acute Pain. IASP Publications, Seattle.

Ready L.B., Oden R., Chadwick H.S. et al. (1988) Development of an anesthesiology-based postoperative pain management service. *Anesthesiology* **68**, 100–106.

Ready L.B., Ashburn M., Caplan R.A. et al. (1995) Practice guidelines for acute pain management in the perioperative setting – a report of the American Society of Anesthesiologists Task Force on Pain Management, Acute Pain Section. *Anesthesiology* **82**, 1071–1081.

Royal College of Surgeons and College of Anaesthetists (1990) Commission on the Provision of Surgical Services. *Report of the Working Party on Pain after Surgery.* London.

Sartain J.B. and Barry J.J. (1999) The impact of an acute pain service in postoperative pain management. *Anaesthesia and Intensive Care* **27**, 375–380.

Stacey B.R., Rudy T.E. and Nellhaus D. (1997) Management of patient-controlled analgesia: a comparison of primary surgeons and a dedicated pain service. *Anesthesia and Analgesia* **85**, 130–134.

Tryba M. (1998) Prevention of chronic pain syndromes by anaesthetic measures: fact or fiction? *Baillière's Clinical Anaesthesiology* **12**, 133–145.

Warfield C.A. and Kahn C.H. (1995) Acute pain management programs in US hospitals and experiences and attitudes among US adults. *Anesthesiology* **83**, 1090–1094.

Weissman C. (1990) The metabolic response to stress: an overview and update. *Anesthesiology* **73**, 308–327.

Wheatley R.J., Madej T.H., Jackson I.J.B. and Hunter D. (1991) The first year's experience of an acute pain service. *British Journal of Anaesthesia* **67**, 353–359.

CHAPTER 2

PHARMACOLOGY OF OPIOIDS

Opioid receptors and endogenous opioids

Effects of opioids

Predictors of opioid dose

Titration of opioid dose

Commonly used opioid agonists

Partial agonists and agonist-antagonists

Opioid antagonists

Opium contains more than 25 different alkaloids. Only two of these have any analgesic action – morphine (10% by weight of opium) and codeine (0.5% by weight). Drugs derived from the alkaloids of opium are called *opiates*. All drugs that have morphine-like actions, naturally occurring or synthetic, are called *opioids*. The term *narcotic*, derived from the Greek word for stupor, is also often used. However, it is probably best confined to a legal context, where it refers to a wide variety of drugs of addiction.

In one of its many forms or preparations, opium has been used for the treatment of pain for over 2000 years. The psychological effects of opium were known to the ancient Sumerians for hundreds of years before that, and reference is made to its analgesic effect in Egyptian mythology. However, the first accepted reference to its use for the treatment of pain is found in the writings of Theophrastus in the third century BC. In 1806 Sertürner isolated the alkaloid of opium later called morphine (after Morpheus – the Greek god of dreams and son of Hypnos, god of sleep). Codeine was isolated in 1832. The introduction of the glass syringe and hollow needle in 1853 enabled the parenteral injection of morphine, facilitating its use and also its abuse.

Morphine is still obtained from the opium poppy, *Papaver somniferum*, as its synthesis is expensive. Traditionally, opium is obtained by incising the unripe seed capsule of the poppy. However, this method of collection is very labor-intensive and an alternative and more modern method of production harvests the dried poppy and extracts morphine, codeine and thebaine from the poppy straw. Morphine remains the standard against which all new analgesics are compared. Although newer opioids may possess special qualities, none is clinically superior in relieving pain. Most of the recent improvements in acute pain management have resulted from the better use of well-established opioids, rather than the use of newer drugs.

OPIOID RECEPTORS AND ENDOGENOUS OPIOIDS

Until the mid-1970s very little was known about the mechanism of action of opioid drugs. Since then, not only have receptor sites for these drugs been identified, but it was also discovered that the body is capable of producing its own (endogenous) opioids.

ENDOGENOUS OPIOIDS

Endogenous opioids identified so far are *endorphins*, *enkephalins* and *dynorphins*. They are found in the brain, spinal cord, gastrointestinal tract and plasma, and are released in response to stimuli such as pain or stress.

Placebo response

Some patients will obtain pain relief from non-analgesic medications or interventions, or a greater than expected degree of relief from an analgesic drug or technique. This is known as the placebo analgesic response and it is though to result, at least in part, from the release of endogenous opioids. The pain relief obtained from nonanalgesic treatment may be partly reversible if the patient is given an opioid antagonist such as naloxone.

OPIOID RECEPTORS

Opioid drugs produce their effect by acting as agonists at opioid receptors, which are found in the brain, spinal cord and sites outside the central nervous system including urinary and gastrointestinal tracts, lung and peripheral nerve endings. There are three principal types of opioid receptor, mu (μ), delta (δ) and kappa (κ). The corresponding endogenous agonists are β-endorphins, enkephalins and dynorphins respectively. A sigma (σ) receptor was initially proposed and thought to mediate the dysphoric and psychotomimetic (hallucinations and delirium) effects of agonist-antagonist opioids. However, these effects are probably the result of κ receptor activity.

A newer classification for opioid receptors has been suggested: OP_1, OP_2 and OP_3 corresponding to δ, κ and μ receptors respectively.

The effects of activation of the different receptors are summarized in **Box 2.1**

According to their action on the opioid receptors, opioid drugs are classed as:

- *agonists:* drugs that bind to and stimulate opioid receptors and are capable of producing a maximal response from the receptor
- *antagonists:* drugs that bind to but do not stimulate opioid receptors and may reverse the effect of opioid agonists

Opioid receptors

Receptor	Action
μ (OP_3)	Analgesia, respiratory depression, euphoria, bradycardia, pruritus, miosis, nausea and vomiting, inhibition of gut motility, physical dependence
δ (OP_1)	Analgesia
κ (OP_2)	Analgesia, sedation, psychotomimetic effects, dysphoria, diuresis

Box 2.1

Possible side effects of opioids	
Respiratory system	Respiratory depression
Central nervous system	Sedation, euphoria (sometimes dysphoria), nausea and vomiting, miosis, muscle rigidity
Cardiovascular system	Vasodilatation, bradycardia, myocardial depression
Genitourinary system	Urinary retention
Gastrointestinal system	Delayed gastric emptying, constipation, spasm of the sphincter of Oddi
Pruritus	Possibly more common with morphine
Allergy	A 'true' allergy is uncommon

Box 2.3

groups have a similar incidence and degree of side effects. However, there may be individual patient differences and some patients may suffer more side effects with one particular drug. In these instances a change to another opioid may be appropriate.

EFFECTS ON THE RESPIRATORY SYSTEM

Opioids affect the respiratory system in a number of ways and can lead to:

- a decrease in respiratory rate
- a decrease in tidal volume
- irregularities in respiratory rhythm, which may lead to periods of hypoventilation and central apnea, particularly when the patient is asleep
- intermittent partial or complete upper airway obstruction (obstructive apnea) when the patient is asleep – see below.

Excessive doses of opioid may result in a progressive clinical respiratory depression; in doses that are not excessive, the last two effects in particular may lead to episodes of intermittent hypoxemia (see below).

Respiratory depression

Respiratory depression is caused by direct action of the drugs on the respiratory center in the brain stem. It is a relatively uncommon (though much feared) complication of opioid administration. All opioids, given in equianalgesic doses, have the same potential for respiratory depression. However, if doses are properly titrated, the risk is very small.

Monitoring respiratory depression – sedation score or respiratory rate?

Traditionally respiratory rate has been used as an indicator of clinical respiratory depression, but a decrease in respiratory rate is now recognized to be a late and unreliable sign. A normal rate may coexist with marked respiratory depression, as inadequate ventilation can result from other opioid-related effects on the respiratory system (upper airway obstruction, a reduction in tidal volume or irregularities in respiratory rhythm).

As respiratory depression is almost always preceded by sedation, the best early clinical indicator of respiratory depression is increasing sedation, which can be monitored using a simple sedation score (**Box 2.4**). When the patient is asleep an assessment can usually be made without fully waking the patient (e.g. the patient turns when the pulse is taken). Opioid doses can be adjusted so that the sedation score remains below 2.

Clinical indicators of respiratory depression

Sedation score	0 = none
	1 = mild, occasionally drowsy, easy to rouse
	2 = moderate, constantly or frequently drowsy (e.g. falls asleep during conversation), easy to rouse
	3 = severe, somnolent, difficult to rouse
	S = normally asleep, easy to rouse
Respiratory rate	Less than 8/min is often considered to indicate respiratory depression but this is generally an unreliable indicator
Oxygen saturation	May also be unreliable, especially, if the patient is receiving supplemental oxygen

Box 2.4

When respiratory rate is counted it should be the unstimulated rate (counted before the patient is roused). In general, a rate of less than 8 breaths per minute is considered to indicate respiratory depression. However, some patients may have rates as low as this or even lower, particularly when asleep, in the absence of respiratory depression. In some centers, respiratory rates of less than 8 per minute are tolerated, as long as the patient is not sedated. As mentioned before, respiratory depression can coexist with a normal respiratory rate.

The administration of sedatives (including benzodiazepines, antihistamines and some antiemetics) will markedly increase the risk of respiratory depression and they should not routinely be given to patients receiving opioids. If sedatives are considered necessary, smaller than normal doses should be used in the first instance. As well as increasing the risk of respiratory depression, the addition of a sedative can make it impossible to give sufficient opioid to achieve patient comfort without causing excessive sedation.

Changes in PO_2, PCO_2 and oxygen saturation with respiratory depression

Oxygen saturation (as measured by pulse oximetry) is used in many wards as an easy and noninvasive measure of blood oxygen levels. However, care must be taken in the interpretation of any readings. If the patient is receiving supplemental oxygen, the added oxygen may mask deterioration in respiratory function (i.e. 'normal' oxygen saturation levels may still be seen). While low oxygen saturation levels in patients receiving oxygen indicate major abnormalities in respiratory function, normal oxygen saturation levels in patients receiving oxygen *do not* exclude abnormalities in respiratory function. In addition, unless continuous oxygen saturation monitoring is used, episodic hypoxemia may be missed.

For example, a healthy young patient before an operation given oxygen at 4 liters per minute may have an arterial PO_2 of 130–150 mmHg (17.3–20 kPa). The pulse oximeter may show an oxygen saturation of 99%. The same patient after a major abdominal operation and receiving the same amount of oxygen may have a PO_2 of only 100 mmHg (13.3 kPa), but the oximeter will show only a small decrease in saturation to 98%. Yet clearly, there is an abnormality in lung function leading to a lesser than expected Po_2 for the inspired oxygen concentration. This would be even more obvious if a patient given oxygen at 10 l/min only had a Po_2 of 100 mmHg (13.3 kPa), far less than would be expected from this inspired oxygen concentration in normal lungs. The oxygen saturation would still be 98% despite obviously abnormal respiratory function.

The relationship between arterial Po_2 and oxygen saturation is not linear, due to the oxygen-hemoglobin dissociation curve (discussed in any physiology textbook). Some approximate values worth remembering are listed in **Box 2.5**.

If arterial blood gas analysis shows an increased arterial Pco_2, regardless of the Po_2 level, opioid-induced respiratory depression should be considered.

Pain antagonizes respiratory depression

Pain is an effective antagonist to opioid-induced respiratory depression. If a patient has received a large dose of opioid as treatment for pain and then, for example, a local anesthetic block is given to manage that pain, onset of the block may be followed by respiratory depression. A similar result may follow if the cause of the pain

Relationship between arterial Po_2 and oxygen saturation

Arterial Po_2 (mmHg)	Arterial Po_2 (kPa)	Oxygen saturation (%)
100	13.3	98
90	12.0	97
80	10.7	95
70	9.3	93
60	8.0	90
40	5.3	75 (venous blood)
26	3.5	50

Box 2.5

is removed. For example, opioids self-administered by a patient using patient-controlled analgesia (PCA) for abdominal pain due to urinary retention may cause respiratory depression when a urinary catheter is inserted and the cause of the pain removed.

Postoperative hypoxemia

Postoperative hypoxemia is reasonably common, especially after major surgery and in the elderly. It can be constant or episodic. In the nonsedated patient, it is most often due to causes other than opioids.

Constant (background) hypoxemia

Reduced lung volumes, particularly vital capacity (VC) and functional residual capacity (FRC), are commonly seen after major surgery. The resultant airways closure, ventilation-perfusion abnormalities and atelectasis, which may be caused by a reduction in FRC, contribute to a constant hypoxemia that may last for a few days. Decreases in FRC peak at 24–48 hours postoperatively and usually resolve within a week. They persist, albeit to a lesser extent, even with complete pain relief. Risk factors for decreased FRC and postoperative hypoxemia include advanced age, upper abdominal and thoracic operations (and to a lesser extent other abdominal operations), obesity, pre-existing lung disease, smoking and severe pain. Patients after major orthopedic (joint replacement) surgery are also likely to be hypoxemic.

Episodic hypoxemia

With normal respiration, an increase in tone of the muscles of the upper airway precedes inspiration and helps maintain airway patency during the negative inspiratory pressures generated by chest and diaphragmatic actions. If the tonic or phasic activity of the upper airway muscles is reduced, as may occur during sleep, closure of the upper airway on inspiration may result. This can manifest as snoring (partial upper airway obstruction) or complete upper airway obstruction (obstructive apnea).

Most obstructive apnea episodes take place during rapid eye movement (REM) sleep, which is also the sleep phase in which most dreaming occurs. Patients who have obstructive sleep apnea (OSA) syndrome may have many obstructive episodes every hour. In the general population the prevalence of OSA is thought to be 5–10%. In the postoperative period, up to 50% of patients may fulfil the criteria for OSA syndrome.

Sleep patterns are often disturbed in the postoperative period or after nonsurgical stress (e.g. severe injury, myocardial infarction). Typically, for the first night or two, there is a reduction in total sleep time, elimination of REM sleep, a reduction in slow wave (very deep non-REM) sleep and increased amounts of lighter non-REM sleep. The disturbance in sleep patterns is greatest after major operations. Rebound REM sleep is typically seen during the second to fourth nights after surgery and is associated with more frequent episodes of airway obstruction than other sleep stages in the postoperative period. Vivid dreams and nightmares are more likely to occur during this increase in REM activity.

Marked reductions in the amount of slow wave sleep and REM sleep may also follow opioid or benzodiazepine administration. In addition, as noted above, any patient given opioids may have episodes of partial or complete airway obstruction when asleep. As with OSA this results from decreased upper airway muscle tone; unlike OSA it can often occur in the absence of REM sleep. This can follow opioid administration by any route and does not necessarily mean that excessive doses of the drug are being given. Patients with OSA are particularly at risk, as are patients given concurrent sedatives.

Any episode of airway obstruction may lead to profound and rapid decreases in oxygen saturation, especially if patients already have a background hypoxemia. Unless continuous pulse oximetry is used, episodic hypoxemia is likely to be missed. Arterial $P\text{CO}_2$ levels may remain within normal limits.

Complications of hypoxemia

Postoperative hypoxemia may lead to cardiac, cerebral and wound complications. Temporal relationships have been shown between episodic hypoxemia and myocardial ischemia, tachycardias and arrhythmias in the postoperative period.

Despite the large number of antiemetic drugs available, PONV remains frustratingly difficult to treat in many patients. The 'perfect' antiemetic agent has yet to be found and in some patients it is only 'tincture of time' that brings any relief.

Antiemetics

There are a number of different classes of antiemetic drugs that act at the different receptor sites involved in the emetic response – dopamine, serotonin (5-hydroxytryptamine or $5HT_3$), acetylcholine (muscarinic type) and histamine.

Antidopaminergic

Several different types of antiemetic drugs have antidopaminergic actions including butyrophenones (e.g. droperidol, haloperidol), phenothiazines (e.g. prochlorperazine) and the gastrointestinal prokinetic drug, metoclopramide.

Droperidol may be as effective as $5HT_3$ inhibitors, depending on factors such as dose used and operation type. The adverse effects of butyrophenones are similar to those of phenothiazines and include extrapyramidal effects (ranging from restlessness and agitation to extrapyramidal reactions including oculogyric crises) and the rare neuroleptic malignant syndrome. Some patients complain of marked apprehension. Lower doses may be as effective in the treatment of PONV as higher doses, but will have a lower incidence of side effects.

Prochlorperazine has been used extensively for many years for the treatment of PONV. Potential side effects are those of any phenothiazine and include extrapyramidal reactions (which may occur after a single dose in some patients).

Metoclopramide acts centrally at dopamine receptors and peripherally to enhance gastric emptying. It also has some antagonistic effects at $5HT_3$ receptor sites. It is probably the most commonly used, albeit the least effective, antiemetic. In most studies it has consistently been shown to be less effective than both $5HT_3$ inhibitors and droperidol, and in some studies little more effective than placebo. Clinically, however, many patients appear to obtain relief and it is widely used in practice. The most important side effects associated with its use are extrapyramidal reactions.

Antiserotinergic

These drugs (e.g. ondansetron, tropisetron and granisetron) inhibit the actions of $5HT_3$ receptors. They are the most effective antiemetics to date. Lack of extrapyramidal side effects and a longer duration of action are advantages; cost is a disadvantage. These drugs are therefore possibly best used as 'rescue' medication when another drug has failed.

Anticholinergic

Scopolamine (hyoscine) has also been used to treat nausea and vomiting. Available as a transdermal patch, and particularly effective for movement-induced nausea and vomiting, it may be associated with significant anticholinergic side effects such as sedation, dry mouth, visual disturbances and confusion.

Antihistamines

Antihistamines such as cyclizine, diphenhydramine, hydroxyzine and promethazine are commonly used as antiemetics and may be particularly effective for movement-induced PONV. Sedation may be a problem.

Steroids

Drugs such as dexamethasone, used in combination with other antiemetic drugs, may also be effective in the treatment of PONV. Such use is not common in current clinical practice.

OTHER EFFECTS ON THE CENTRAL NERVOUS SYSTEM
Miosis, sedation, euphoria and muscle rigidity

Opioids cause constriction of the pupils (miosis) and sedation, but it is important to remember that sedation may precede respiratory depression. While a mild euphoria may be associated with opioid administration, dysphoria and hallucinations occur occasionally. Muscle rigidity has been reported following doses of opioid much larger than those routinely used in pain management.

Pruritus does not always require treatment. If the itching disturbs the patient, the safest treatment in the first instance is to change drugs (e.g. from morphine to fentanyl). Antihistamines (especially parenteral antihistamines) may add to the risk of sedation and respiratory depression. Pruritus may also respond to small, carefully titrated doses of intravenous naloxone. There is, however, a risk that naloxone will reverse the analgesia, although this is less likely if given following the administration of an epidural or intrathecal opioid. Intravenous nalbuphine, in small doses, is also effective in some cases. The $5HT_3$ antagonist ondansetron has been used to treat pruritus in some patients, as has the anesthetic drug propofol.

Allergy

Patients and staff alike will often mistakenly report any adverse reaction to a drug as an allergy (e.g. nausea and vomiting following the administration of opioids; gastrointestinal upsets following the use of antibiotics). True allergic reactions to opioids are mediated by the immune system and result in signs and symptoms that are similar to other allergic reactions including rash, urticaria, bronchoconstriction, angioneurotic edema and cardiovascular disturbances.

PREDICTORS OF OPIOID DOSE

Traditionally the dose of opioid prescribed for a patient has been based – if indeed it was based on anything – on the weight of the patient. In fact there is no clinically significant correlation between patient weight and opioid requirement. The best clinical predictor of opioid dose is patient age. **Figure 2.1** shows the average intravenous PCA morphine requirements of 1010 opioid-naive patients in the first 24 hours after major surgery. The total amount of morphine used in 24 hours decreases significantly as patient age increases. From **Figure 2.1** it can be seen that the average first 24-hour morphine requirements were about 80 mg, 54 mg and 36 mg for patients aged 20 years, 45 years and 70 years respectively. If a straight line is drawn through points

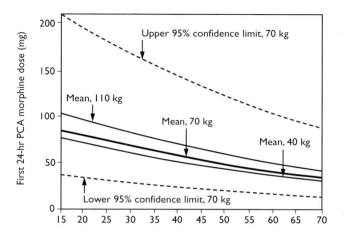

Figure 2.1 First 24-hour PCA morphine requirements and patient age. Adapted with permission from Macintyre and Jarvis (1996)

representing 80 mg, 55 mg and 30 mg for these age groups (and the difference from the original points is well within the differences due to interpatient variation in each age group), it can be seen that after the age of 20 years, first 24-hour morphine requirements decrease by about 1 mg for each additional year of age, or:

average first 24-hour morphine requirements (mg) for patients over 20 years of age = 100 − (age in years)

Note the enormous variation (eightfold to tenfold) in dose requirements in each age group. This means that although the initial dose of opioid should be based on the age of the patient, subsequent doses still need to be titrated to effect for each patient.

Although the weight of the patient has some effect on dose it is clinically insignificant in comparison to the overall interpatient variation.

There are a number of reasons why the dose of opioid required for pain relief should change with patient age. These include age-related changes in pharmacokinetics (how the individual handles the drug, e.g. drug distribution, metabolism and elimination) and pharmacodynamics (how the individual responds to the drug, e.g. perception of pain).

TITRATION OF OPIOID DOSE

For an opioid to be effective it must reach a certain blood level (this applies to parenterally and enterally administered opioids and not to epidural and intrathecal opioids, which are discussed in Chapter 6). The effective range of blood concentrations varies some fourfold to fivefold between patients. The amount of opioid that each patient requires will also vary according to the severity of the pain stimulus. Thus titration of opioids is needed in order to individualize treatment.

The lowest concentration of opioid that will produce analgesia is known as the *minimum effective analgesic concentration* (MEAC). Below this level a patient will experience no pain relief and above it there will be increasing analgesia and an increasing possibility of side effects. In reality the boundaries are somewhat blurred and side effects may occur before good pain relief is obtained. The therapeutic range of blood levels (where analgesia is achieved without significant side effects) is often colloquially referred to as the 'analgesic corridor' (**Figure 2.2**). For each patient the aim of titration is to find and then maintain the effective blood level within this 'corridor'. A change in pain intensity may shift the corridor and require an increase or decrease in opioid dose.

To enable opioid analgesia to be titrated for each patient, appropriate doses and dose intervals need to be ordered. In addition, endpoints that indicate adequate or excessive doses need to be monitored repeatedly.

DOSE RANGE

The range of doses prescribed should center on the average for the age of the patient and will vary according to the route of administration of the drug.

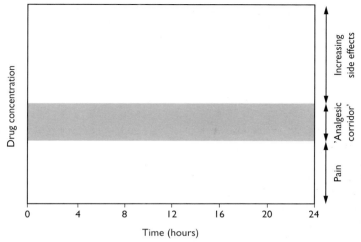

Figure 2.2 'Analgesic corridor'

DOSE INTERVAL

When an interval is prescribed between intermittent doses of opioid, the aim of the interval is primarily to allow the full effect of the previous dose to be seen before another dose may be given. It is also often used to give an indication of the expected duration of action of the drug.

The speed of onset of effect of an opioid will be influenced by its route of administration and its lipid solubility. The time taken for an opioid to reach a maximum blood concentration depends primarily on the route of administration. However, the time taken to then achieve maximum effect depends on the rate at which the drug crosses to the central nervous system and opioid receptors. Factors that determine the rate of this transfer include the lipid solubility of the drug (**Box 2.6**) and the concentration gradient. Of the opioids in common clinical use, morphine is the least lipid-soluble and has the longest delay. It may take up to 15 minutes or more following an intravenous injection for its maximum effect to be seen. The full effect of intravenous fentanyl, on the other hand, may be seen within 5 minutes.

Lipid solubilities of some of the commonly used opioids

Opioid	Lipid solubility*
Morphine	1
Meperidine (pethidine)	39
Fentanyl	813
Alfentanil	129
Sufentanil	1780
Diamorphine	280
Methadone	116
Hydromorphone	1.4

Box 2.6
*Octanol/pH 7.4 buffer partition coefficient.
Values may vary according to different references.

Although less lipid-soluble than fentanyl, the maximum effect of alfentanil may be seen within 1–2 minutes. This is because of the much greater proportion of alfentanil present in a nonionized form. The time to peak effect needs to be taken into account when dose intervals are prescribed.

The duration of action of any given dose of opioid also depends on a number of factors including the amount given, the route of administration, and pharmacokinetic characteristics of the drug such as absorption, rate of distribution to different tissues (including receptors), rate of dissociation from receptors, lipid solubility and elimination half-life $(t_{\frac{1}{2}\beta})$. The elimination half-life alone does not determine duration of action. It is the time taken for the blood concentration of the drug to change by 50%, and gives an indication of the rate at which the body metabolizes and excretes the drug.

Drugs are metabolized to a form that is more easily excreted. In the case of opioids, the liver is the primary site of metabolism and the kidney the primary route of excretion of metabolites. The metabolites of some opioids have analgesic and other effects.

MONITORING OF PAIN AND SEDATION SCORES AND OTHER SIDE EFFECTS

When titrating any drug, ongoing monitoring of endpoints that indicate 'how much is enough' and 'how much is too much' is needed. The best way to monitor the former is to use a pain score and functional assessment. The most serious consequence of excessive opioid dose is respiratory depression and, as outlined before, the best early indication of this is sedation, although respiratory rate is usually also counted. Nausea and vomiting or lightheadedness may also indicate a slightly excessive dose.

The aim of pain treatment is to make the patient comfortable while keeping the sedation score below 2 (**Box 2.7**). If the patient does become sedated, subsequent doses should be reduced. If the patient is uncomfortable and not sedated, a larger dose may be required. Although many guidelines suggest that the respiratory rate should be maintained at above 8 breaths per minute, there may be occasions when a lower rate can be tolerated provided the patient is not sedated.

Some concurrent medical conditions or medications may affect the metabolism or excretion of opioids and their metabolites. It is not possible to predict the degree of impairment from alterations in laboratory tests of renal or hepatic function,

Titration of opioids

Requirements:
- an age-related range of doses
- dose intervals appropriate to the route of administration
- monitoring of pain score, sedation score and respiratory rate
- monitoring for presence of other side effects

Aims:
- patient comfort
- sedation score < 2, respiratory rate > 8/min (in most cases)

Box 2.7

but careful titration will allow the appropriate adjustments in dose and dose interval to be made.

COMMONLY USED OPIOID AGONISTS

These drugs are primarily μ receptor agonists.

MORPHINE

Morphine is the least lipid-soluble of all opioids in common use. It is metabolized principally in the liver and less than 10% is excreted unchanged by the kidneys.

The main metabolites of morphine, morphine 6-glucuronide (M6G) and morphine 3-glucuronide (M3G), have longer half-lives than morphine and are primarily excreted via the kidney. Morphine 6-glucuronide is a more potent μ receptor agonist than morphine and may contribute significantly to its analgesic effect, particularly in patients on long-term morphine therapy. It also has the same spectrum of side effects as morphine. In patients with reduced renal function the half-life of morphine is not significantly increased. However, there may be an apparent prolongation of its effect due to accumulation of M6G.

Morphine 3-glucuronide has no analgesic activity and does not appear to compete for opioid receptor binding sites. It may even antagonize the analgesic effects of morphine and M6G, although this is not yet clear. There is some evidence that M3G may influence the development of morphine tolerance and that it might be responsible for some of the side effects seen with long-term, high-dose morphine treatment, such as myoclonus, hyperalgesia and allodynia.

Morphine can be given by intramuscular, intravenous, subcutaneous, oral, transmucosal, rectal, epidural and intrathecal routes. Dose ranges and dose intervals will vary according to the route of administration.

Slow- or sustained-release preparations of oral morphine are available for the treatment of chronic and cancer pain and only need to be given two or three times a day. The slower onset (3–4 hours or longer) and prolonged duration of action of these formulations make fast titration of the drug impossible, so these preparations are usually unsuitable for the treatment of acute pain, at least in the initial stages.

PAPAVERETUM

Like opium, papaveretum contains a mixture of opium alkaloids. The percentage of morphine by weight is 50%. Although a popular choice of drug in Britain and Australia, there is no advantage in using this preparation compared with using morphine alone.

CODEINE

Codeine is a naturally occurring alkaloid like morphine. It is metabolized in the liver where about 10% of the dose is converted to morphine. This probably accounts for most of the analgesic effect of codeine, as the drug itself has a very low affinity for opioid receptors. Metabolism to morphine involves the enzyme CYP2D6. This enzyme is part of the cytochrome P450 system and may not be present in all people. Eight to ten per cent of the white population are thought to lack this enzyme and these patients will obtain little or no pain relief from codeine.

Codeine is usually given for the treatment of mild to moderate pain by intramuscular or oral routes. There are a number of oral formulations that combine codeine with non-opioid analgesics such as acetaminophen (paracetamol) or aspirin.

DIAMORPHINE (HEROIN)

Diamorphine does not bind to opioid receptors and has no analgesic activity. It is a *prodrug* and is rapidly hydrolyzed to 6-monoacetylmorphine (a potent analgesic) and then morphine. It has not been shown to have any clinical advantage over morphine when administered by oral or intramuscular routes. Both diamorphine and 6-monoacetylmorphine are more lipid-soluble than morphine; diamorphine therefore has a more rapid onset of action when given by intravenous or epidural routes. Diamorphine is not available for medical use in Australia or the USA.

OXYCODONE

Oxycodone is a thebaine derivative. Because it was first introduced into some countries in oral formulations combined with acetaminophen (paracetamol) or aspirin, it was considered suitable for the treatment of mild to moderate pain only. It is the limitations placed on the total dose of acetaminophen or aspirin that can be given to a patient in any one day that may limit the usefulness of the combined formulations. Like all pure opioid agonists there is no ceiling effect to analgesia and in higher doses oxycodone can be used for the treatment of severe pain.

The major metabolite of oxycodone is noroxycodone, which has much less analgesic activity. It is renally excreted. Oxymorphone, another metabolite, possesses significant analgesic activity. However, it is present only in very low concentrations and contributes little to the pain-relieving effect of oxycodone. The formation of oxymorphone depends on the enzyme CYP2D6 (see codeine above).

Oxycodone can be given by parenteral, oral and rectal routes. A slow-release formulation of oral oxycodone is now available. It may have a quicker onset of action compared with currently available slow-release morphine preparations.

MEPERIDINE (PETHIDINE)

Meperidine was first synthesized just prior to World War II as a potential substitute for atropine. In addition to its analgesic effect, meperidine has some atropine-like actions that may lead to a dry mouth or slight tachycardia, and some local anesthetic activity (this latter effect has allowed intrathecal meperidine to be used as the sole agent for spinal anesthesia). Myocardial depression can occur with larger doses. In patients taking monoamine oxidase inhibitors, hyperpyrexia, convulsions, coma and hypertension or hypotension have been reported following the administration of meperidine. Meperidine is thought to have a weak affinity for the N-methyl-D-aspartate (NMDA), receptor (see Chapter 7).

Meperidine can be given by intramuscular or intravenous injection or infusion (subcutaneous injections may be excessively painful) as well as by oral, rectal, transmucosal, epidural and intrathecal routes. Like morphine, the range of doses and dose durations required will vary according to the route of administration.

Unlike other opioids, meperidine has been used to treat shivering associated with volatile anesthetic agents, epidural and spinal anesthesia, and chemotherapy. The usual initial dose is 12–25 mg IV.

Meperidine is primarily metabolized in the liver and the metabolites excreted by the kidney. Less than 10% of meperidine is excreted unchanged by the kidneys. One of the main metabolites is normeperidine (norpethidine) which has a long half-life of 15–20 hours. A build-up of this metabolite can lead to normeperidine toxicity.

Normeperidine (norpethidine) toxicity

Normeperidine is a μ agonist and therefore analgesic, but it also has other nonopioid effects. High blood levels can lead to signs of central nervous system (CNS) excitation including anxiety, mood change, tremors, twitching, myoclonic jerks and even frank convulsions (**Box 2.8**). Patients receiving large doses of meperidine or those with renal impairment are particularly at risk.

Signs of normeperidine toxicity can be seen within 24–36 hours in some healthy and young patients with normal renal function who require doses in the higher range for each age group. It was probably not seen in this group of patients until recently because very few would have been given more than 100 mg meperidine 4-hourly – a total of only 600 mg a day. With the advent of PCA, patients can receive much higher doses and therefore normeperidine levels will rise more rapidly.

There is no specific treatment for normeperidine toxicity. Meperidine should be discontinued and another opioid substituted. Naloxone should not be given, as it will antagonize the sedative effect of meperidine but not the excitatory effects of normeperidine. It will therefore only exacerbate the problem.

As there is no specific treatment it is important to watch for early signs and symptoms of toxicity and prevent excessive levels of normeperidine by limiting the amount of meperidine

Normeperidine (norpethidine) toxicity

Effects of normeperidine	analgesia (μ receptor mediated)
	CNS excitation (nonopioid effect)
Half-life ($t_{\frac{1}{2}\beta}$)	15–20 hours
Signs and symptoms	Anxiety, agitation, mood change, tremors,
	twitching, myoclonic jerks, convulsions
Treatment	Discontinue meperidine
	Substitute an alternative opioid
	Symptomatic treatment of effects
	DO NOT administer naloxone
Dose limits (suggested)	1000 mg in first 24 hours
	600–700 mg/day thereafter
	These dose limits should be reduced in the
	elderly or in patients with renal impairment

Box 2.8

administered. It is difficult to predict exactly what dose of meperidine or what blood level of normeperidine is likely to cause normeperidine toxicity in any particular patient. However, it is suggested that young patients with normal renal function should not receive more than 1000 mg in the first 24 hours of treatment. Subsequent totals should probably not exceed 600–700 mg per 24 hours. These limits should be reduced for elderly patients and patients with renal impairment.

METHADONE

A synthetic opioid developed during World War II, methadone has a much longer half-life than other opioids and therefore a much longer duration of action. This makes fast titration with methadone more difficult than with shorter half-life drugs. Methadone is more commonly used for the management of chronic pain or in drug dependency treatment programs. It can be given by oral, intravenous, intramuscular and epidural routes.

Single doses of methadone may produce a quality and duration of analgesia similar to a single equianalgesic dose of morphine (See **Box 2.2**). However, the long half-life of methadone means that significant accumulation of drug can occur. Total daily dose requirements are therefore not comparable. If a patient has been taking another opioid for some time and changes to methadone, methadone doses should start at about 10% of the calculated equianalgesic dose and be titrated to effect.

Methadone is thought to be an NMDA receptor antagonist (see Chapter 7) and may be of use in the treatment of neuropathic pain (see Chapter 10).

HYDROMORPHONE

A semisynthetic opioid (a direct derivative of morphine), hydromorphone is available in oral, parenteral and suppository forms and can also be used for epidural analgesia.

FENTANYL AND ITS ANALOGS

Fentanyl is a highly lipid-soluble synthetic opioid that does not cause histamine release. It has a more rapid onset of action than morphine and single doses have a short duration of action because of rapid tissue uptake from plasma. The metabolites of fentanyl are inactive and therefore fentanyl is a good choice of opioid in patients with renal impairment.

For the treatment of acute pain fentanyl can be administered intravenously (for example, by PCA), epidurally or intrathecally. Oral transmucosal ('lollipop') administration has been used in children; true oral administration is not suitable because of the very high first pass effect. The high lipid solubility of fentanyl makes it suitable for transdermal administration, but recently developed transdermal delivery systems for fentanyl (see Chapter 4) have not proved successful for the management of acute pain.

Alfentanil and sufentanil are both highly lipid-soluble. They have a more rapid onset and shorter duration of action than fentanyl, despite the lower lipid solubility of alfentanil. This makes them very suitable for administration by intravenous infusion during anesthesia, but probably of limited use in the postoperative period. They have been used either alone, or in combination with local anesthetics agents, for epidural analgesia. Both drugs are primarily eliminated by the liver.

A newer opioid, remifentanil, has very rapid onset. It also has an ultra-short duration of action owing to its metabolism by nonspecific blood and tissue esterases. It is mainly used in clinical practice as an infusion during anesthesia. Depending on the type of surgery, postoperative pain may be significant unless postoperative analgesic strategies are introduced before stopping the remifentanil infusion.

TRAMADOL

Tramadol is a centrally acting synthetic analgesic. It has some μ-opioid receptor activity (thought to account for about 30–50% of its analgesic action) and it inhibits the reuptake of norepineph-rine (noradrenaline) and serotonin (5-hydroxytryptamine, 5HT) at nerve terminals. This latter action is similar to the mechanism of action of tricyclic antidepressants (see Chapter 10).

The advantages over other opioids are said to be an absence of tolerance, a lower abuse potential (it is not a controlled drug), and less respiratory depression, although some reports cast doubt on these claims. There may be less constipation. When used for postoperative analgesia, nausea, vomiting and sedation may still occur. A history of epilepsy may be a contraindication to its use, as convulsions have been reported.

Tramadol is available in oral and parenteral forms. As bioavailability following oral administration is high, doses are similar for both oral and parenteral routes. Product information sheets may suggest a total daily dose ceiling of about 600 mg. This will limit the usefulness of tramadol in the treatment of severe acute pain. Tramadol may also be given by the epidural route.

As the opioid receptor effects of the drug are relatively weak, it may not be suitable as the sole analgesic in patients who are opioid-dependent.

The main metabolite of tramadol is O-desmethyltramadol (M1), which has analgesic activity. It is more potent than tramadol and may contribute to its analgesic efficacy. The formation of M1 depends on the enzyme CYP2D6 (see codeine above). Further metabolism results in inactive compounds that are excreted by the kidney.

OTHER OPIOIDS

The opioids listed below are commonly available as an oral formulation combined with a non-opioid analgesic, which limits the amount of the opioid that can be given.

Propoxyphene

Structurally similar to methadone, only the dextrorotatory (R isomer) form has any analgesic activity (dextropropoxyphene). Often administered in an oral formulation in combination with acetaminophen (paracetamol) or aspirin, these preparations may be no more effective than acetaminophen or aspirin alone. Toxicity, with hallucinations, delusions and confusion, may occur with accumulation of the renally excreted active metabolite norpropoxyphene, but this is unlikely to be significant at doses used clinically. The $t_{\frac{1}{2}\beta}$ is 6–12 hours. It is thought to be a weak NMDA receptor antagonist (see Chapter 7).

Hydrocodone

Hydrocodone is available in the USA only in combination formulations with non-opioid analgesics such as acetaminophen. Its $t_{\frac{1}{2}\beta}$ is similar to codeine.

PARTIAL AGONISTS AND AGONIST-ANTAGONISTS

Buprenorphine is usually classed as a partial agonist while the other drugs listed below are agonist-antagonists. Agonist-antagonist drugs derive their analgesic actions principally from κ receptor activation while acting as antagonists at the μ receptor. When given in doses that are equianalgesic to morphine, these drugs result in the same side effects although (unlike pure agonists) there is a ceiling effect for both analgesia and respiratory depression. Respiratory depression has, however, been reported. The agonist-antagonist opioids are associated with a higher incidence of dysphoria and sedation than pure agonist opioids.

These drugs are said to have a lower potential for abuse than other opioids, but this is of limited significance in patients with no previous history of substance abuse and in whom the risk of addiction to opioids used for the treatment of acute pain is minimal. The agonist-antagonist drugs can precipitate withdrawal signs and symptoms in opioid-dependent patients.

On the whole, partial agonist and agonist-antagonist opioid drugs are used far less commonly in clinical practice than the pure opioid agonist drugs.

BUPRENORPHINE
Buprenorphine is derived from the opium alkaloid thebaine and is available in parenteral and sublingual formulations. It is highly lipid-soluble, hence its excellent absorption by the sublingual route. It dissociates slowly from the μ receptor and therefore duration of action may be prolonged. Dysphoric side effects are relatively uncommon; other side effects are similar to morphine.

PENTAZOCINE
Pentazocine was the first drug of this class to become established in clinical practice. It can be given orally or parenterally. The high incidence of dysphoria associated with the drug has limited its use.

NALBUPHINE
Chemically related to naloxone, nalbuphine is available as a parenteral preparation. It may be effective in reversing some of the side effects of μ-agonist drugs, such as respiratory depression and pruritus.

BUTORPHANOL
Butorphanol is available as parenteral and intranasal preparations.

OPIOID ANTAGONISTS

These drugs are antagonists at all receptor sites; the most commonly used is naloxone.

NALOXONE

The $t_{\frac{1}{2}\beta}$ of naloxone, about 60 minutes, is much shorter than that of the drugs listed above. As a result, if naloxone is required to antagonize the effects of most opioid agonists, repeated doses or an infusion may be needed. By titrating the dose of naloxone, it is possible to reverse opioid-related respiratory depression, excessive sedation, nausea and vomiting, and pruritus, while still retaining reasonable analgesia. However, this balance may be more difficult to obtain when opioids are being administered by other than epidural or intrathecal routes.

For the treatment of respiratory depression and excessive sedation, 40–100 micrograms of naloxone should be given intravenously and repeated every few minutes as required. If there is no venous access available, naloxone can be given in larger doses (e.g. 400 µg) by subcutaneous or intramuscular injection. Smaller doses may be more suitable if naloxone is used to reverse other side effects of opioids. If a patient is on chronic opioid therapy, it is especially important to titrate naloxone in order to avoid precipitation of withdrawal signs and symptoms.

While some cardiovascular stimulation (hypertension, tachycardia) or nausea and vomiting may be seen after administration of naloxone, especially after rapid reversal of analgesia, serious side effects such as pulmonary edema and arrhythmias are rare.

Naloxone is poorly absorbed following oral administration but has been used for treatment of opioid-induced constipation.

NALTREXONE

Unlike naloxone, naltrexone is effective when given orally. It has a half-life of 2–4 hours and its main metabolite is 6-naltrexol, a weaker µ opioid antagonist but with a half-life of more than 8 hours. Naltrexone has been used in the treatment of opioid addiction where the effects of a 50 mg dose may last up to 24

CHAPTER 3

PHARMACOLOGY OF LOCAL ANESTHETIC DRUGS

Mechanism of action

Adverse effects of local anesthetic drugs

Classes of local anesthetic drugs

Commonly used local anesthetic drugs

Equieffective anesthetic concentrations

Cocaine was first introduced into medical practice in 1884 by Koller, who described its use for topical anesthesia of the cornea. This was followed by its use in nerve conduction blockade and local infiltration anesthesia. In 1899 Bier reported on the application of cocaine in spinal anesthesia.

The toxicity of cocaine and its brief duration of action limited its usefulness in surgical practice and led to a search for less toxic substances. The synthesis of procaine by Einhorn in 1905 and lidocaine (lignocaine) by Löfgren and Lundqvist in 1943 heralded the development of local anesthetic drugs in common use today.

MECHANISM OF ACTION

Local anesthetic drugs block transmission of nerve impulses within the central nervous system (CNS). The generation and propagation of a nerve impulse along a nerve fiber involves the opening of sodium channels in the nerve membrane and the massive flow of sodium ions from the outside to the inside of the membrane. Local anesthetic drugs prevent the influx of sodium ions, thereby blocking conduction of the nerve impulse.

There are a number of different types of nerve fibers and these vary in size and function (**Box 3.1**).

It is commonly believed that smaller-diameter nerve fibers are more easily blocked than those with a larger diameter, but diameter is not important. The ease with which a nerve fiber is blocked by a local anesthetic drug depends on its *critical blocking length* (the length that must be exposed to the drug in order for the nerve to become blocked) and the *accessibility* of nerve membrane binding sites to the blocking agent.

However, smaller-diameter fibers have the smallest critical blocking lengths and are more easily accessed and blocked by local anesthetic solutions. Nerve blockade is also *frequency dependent* – active nerve fibers are more easily blocked than inactive ones.

The onset and regression of a nerve block usually progresses according to the order in **Box 3.2** but this may vary a little between patients and different drugs. Note that B fibers tend to be blocked before C fibers. This is probably because C fibers are usually arranged in Remak bundles, which may hamper diffusion of local anesthetic solutions, and/or because the critical blocking length of B fibers is quite short.

As the effect of a nerve block is wearing off, recovery of movement (larger fibers) may precede recovery of sensation or

Nerve fiber class, size and function

Class	Size	Function
A-alpha (Aα)	Largest	Motor, proprioception (position sense)
A-beta (Aβ)		Touch, pressure
A-gamma (Aγ)		Muscle spindle tone
A-delta (Aδ)		Pain, temperature, touch
B		Preganglionic autonomic (sympathetic)
C (unmyelinated)	Smallest	Pain/temperature
		Postganglionic autonomic (sympathetic)

Box 3.1

Onset and recovery of nerve block according to fiber size		
	Order of onset	*Order of recovery*
First	B	Aα
	C, Aδ	Aβ
	Aγ	Aγ
	Aβ	Aδ, C
Last	Aα	B

Box 3.2

sympathetic nerve function (smaller fibers). This is of particular importance following epidural or spinal anesthesia, when a patient may appear to have normal motor function yet may have incomplete return of sensation, and a residual sympathetic block that could lead to postural (orthostatic) hypotension.

Epidural analgesia is commonly employed as a method of postoperative pain relief. Low concentrations of local anesthetic drug are often used in an attempt to block sensory fibers only (*differential nerve block*). This means that the patient may be able to move and walk normally while still receiving good pain relief. However, this cannot be assumed and every patient should be assessed before walking is allowed. Note that while there is analgesia, blockade of sympathetic nerve fibers may be present and postural hypotension remains a potential risk.

ADVERSE EFFECTS OF LOCAL ANESTHETIC DRUGS

The adverse effects that may follow administration of a local anesthetic agent can be a result of the physiological effects of the nerves blocked, local tissue toxicity or systemic toxicity.

PHYSIOLOGICAL EFFECTS

Physiological effects are most common following epidural and spinal anesthesia or analgesia and are covered in Chapter 6.

LOCAL TISSUE TOXICITY

The local anesthetic agents in common clinical use rarely produce localized nerve damage. However, all are capable of causing nerve injury when used in sufficiently high concentrations. Motor and sensory nerve deficits following subarachnoid administration of chloroprocaine were reported and thought to be due to the presence of the antioxidant, sodium bisulfite, in the solution. The sodium bisulfite was replaced with ethylenediaminetetraacetic acid (EDTA) in later formulations but reports of back pain have occurred. Intrathecal hyperbaric 5% lidocaine solutions appear to have a higher potential for local neurotoxicity compared with other concentrations and other local anesthetic drugs commonly used for spinal anesthesia.

SYSTEMIC TOXICITY

High blood concentrations of local anesthetic drugs can lead to signs and symptoms of systemic toxicity. This can occur if excessive doses of local anesthetic agent are given, or if an otherwise safe dose is inadvertently injected directly into a blood vessel. Systemic toxicity results from the effects of local anesthetic drugs on the CNS and cardiovascular system. The higher the blood concentration the more severe the signs and symptoms (**Box 3.3**). Not all the signs and symptoms will necessarily occur in every patient.

A number of factors will influence the blood concentrations of local anesthetic agent reached after injection:

- *dose of drug:* this should be appropriate for the patient and the local block procedure employed; 'recommended' or 'safe' doses may be excessive if injected directly into blood vessels or tissues with a rich vascular supply
- *site of injection:* the rate of absorption of local anesthetic agents depends to a large extent on the blood supply to the area; the order, from most to least rapid, is interpleural > intercostal > caudal > epidural > brachial plexus > sciatic/femoral
- *vasoconstrictor:* with some local anesthetic drugs (short to medium duration, e.g. lidocaine and mepivacaine) the addition of a vasoconstrictor such as epinephrine (adrenaline) will decrease the rate of absorption of drug into

Signs and symptoms of systemic local anesthetic toxicity

Cardiovascular depression
Respiratory arrest
Coma
Convulsions
Unconsciousness
Drowsiness
Muscular twitching
Tinnitus, visual disturbances
Circumoral numbness and numbness of tongue
Lightheadedness

↑ *Increasing blood concentrations*

Box 3.3

the circulation, prolonging duration of action and leading to lower blood levels for the same dose; little if any effect is seen if epinephrine is added to bupivacaine or ropivacaine

- *speed of injection*: the more rapid the rate of injection the more rapid the rise in plasma concentration of the drug; in a general ward a continuous infusion of local anesthetic solution may be the safest method of administration
- *metabolism of the drug*

Central nervous system toxicity

Signs and symptoms of CNS toxicity are generally seen at lower blood concentrations than those leading to cardiovascular toxicity. The early signs are those of CNS excitation, due to initial blockade of inhibitory pathways. These are best detected by maintaining verbal contact with the patient who, as blood concentrations of the drug rise, may complain of numbness around the mouth and tongue, a feeling of lightheadedness, and ringing in the ears. Slurring of speech and muscle twitching will follow and the patient may become drowsy. If the blood level continues to rise a generalized convulsion (usually brief) will occur and at even higher blood concentrations respiratory depression and arrest will ensue.

ESTERS

Cocaine

Cocaine has a number of actions in addition to its ability to block conduction of nerve impulses. It causes general stimulation of the CNS and blocks reuptake of catecholamines at adrenergic nerve endings, thus potentiating the effects of sympathetic nervous system stimulation. These changes can lead to euphoria and a feeling of wellbeing, restlessness, excitement, tachycardia, peripheral vasoconstriction, hypertension, arrhythmias, myocardial ischemia and convulsions. Because of its potential for toxicity, cocaine is now restricted to use as a topical anesthetic agent, usually in surgery involving the nose or preceding nasal endotracheal intubation, where its local vasoconstrictor effect helps to shrink nasal mucosa and reduce bleeding. Doses should be kept within recommended limits to avoid the risk of side effects.

Tetracaine (amethocaine)

Like dibucaine, tetracaine is primarily used for spinal anesthesia.

Procaine

Procaine was the first synthetic local anesthetic agent introduced into clinical practice. Its use is now confined mainly to local infiltration.

Chloroprocaine

Because of its rapid onset, rapid metabolism and short duration of action, chloroprocaine has been primarily used in obstetric epidural analgesia or regional anesthetic techniques for day surgery. Neurotoxicity, with motor and sensory deficits, has followed accidental subarachnoid injection; the sodium bisulfite antioxidant in the anesthetic solution was implicated. The bisulfite has been replaced by EDTA in later formulations but this has been followed by reports of muscle spasm and backache.

EQUIEFFECTIVE ANESTHETIC CONCENTRATIONS

Just as opioids have equianalgesic doses, local anesthetic drugs given in equal volumes have equieffective anesthetic concentrations (**Box 3.5**). Total dose is also an important determinant of effect.

Equieffective anesthetic concentrations

Local anesthetic drug	Concentration (%)
Chloroprocaine	2
Procaine	2
Bupivacaine	0.25
Lidocaine (lignocaine)	1
Ropivacaine	0.25–0.35*
Mepivacaine	1
Etidocaine	0.5
Prilocaine	1

Box 3.5
*Results vary according to different studies.

REFERENCES AND FURTHER READING

Covino B.J. and Wildsmith J.A.W. (1998) Clinical pharmacology of local anesthetic agents. In *Neural Blockade in Clinical Anesthesia and Management of Pain* (eds Cousins M.J. and Bridenbaugh P.O.). Lippincott-Raven Publishers, Philadelphia.

De Jong R.H. (1994) *Local Anesthetics*. Mosby, St Louis.

Liu S.S. (1998) Local anesthetics and analgesia. In *The Management of Pain* (eds Ashburn M.A. and Rice L.J.). Churchill Livingstone, Philadelphia.

McClure J.H. (1996) Ropivacaine. *British Journal of Anaesthesia* **76**, 300–307.

Rosenberg P.H. (1994) Clinical pharmacology and applications of local anesthetics. In *The Pharmacologic Basis of Anesthesiology* (eds Bowdle T.A., Horita A. and Kharasch E.D.). Churchill Livingstone, New York.

CHAPTER 4

ROUTES OF OPIOID ADMINISTRATION

Intramuscular administration

Intermittent subcutaneous administration

Oral administration

Intermittent intravenous administration

Continuous intravenous infusions

Rectal administration

Transdermal administration

Transmucosal administration

Peripheral administration

(For spinal administration of opioids see Chapter 6)

The introduction of more sophisticated methods for the administration of opioids, such as patient-controlled and epidural analgesia, has undoubtedly improved the management of acute pain. However, the more traditional and conventional methods of administration remain in common use, even in centers where the more advanced techniques are available. Studies continue to show that use of these methods frequently results in inadequate analgesia, yet only a few attempts have been made to improve their effectiveness.

Lasagna and Beecher (1954) considered the 'optimal' dose of morphine that should be given by subcutaneous (SC) injection for the relief of postoperative pain. After comparing doses of 10 mg and 15 mg, and because the latter dose had a higher incidence of side effects, they wrote that 'the optimal dose appears to be 10 mg per 70 kg of body weight.' They correctly defined 'optimal dose' as the dose that would give maximum therapeutic effect with minimum adverse effect. However, they unfortunately also cautioned against flexibility in dosing because of the risk of 'dangerous' side effects, and advised against high doses because of the 'known' risk of addiction with larger doses.

That teaching has changed little over the intervening years. It makes no allowances for the enormous interpatient variation in opioid requirements (eightfold to tenfold) that result from the unpredictable differences in pharmacokinetic factors (how the individual patient handles the drug – i.e. how it is absorbed, distributed, metabolized and excreted) and pharmacodynamic factors (how the individual responds to the drug). The same dose of opioid given to different patients can result in a fourfold to fivefold difference in peak blood levels reached; the peak blood concentration from the same dose of opioid may vary twofold within the same patient; and there is a fourfold to fivefold interpatient variation in the minimum effective analgesic concentration (MEAC). Added to this has been the lack of appropriate education of medical and nursing staff, unfounded fears about the risks of side effects and addiction, and a lack of assessment of pain and the results (or otherwise) of its treatment.

It is hardly surprising that traditional regimens for pain relief have been less than successful. However, to a large extent, this is a consequence of deficiencies in their application rather than limitations associated with the route of administration.

The key to making these methods more effective is to individualize opioid treatment regimens for each patient. Effectiveness of analgesia and possible side effects need to be monitored regularly and dose and frequency of administration altered accordingly, so that each drug, regardless of route of administration, is titrated to suit each patient. The introduction of education programs for medical and nursing staff and simple guidelines for techniques such as intermittent intravenous (IV), intramuscular (IM) or SC opioid injections (which include treatment algorithms and regular monitoring of pain) can lead to significant improvements in pain relief. It is also important to allow the patient, where possible, some input into the size of the dose and the timing of each dose. 'Patient control' should not be confined to PCA pump systems.

INTRAMUSCULAR ADMINISTRATION

Although morphine was first given by SC injection, the IM route has become the more common route of administration in the belief (somewhat mistaken) that absorption is slower from subcutaneous sites.

Traditionally, IM opioids have been ordered 4-hourly PRN (*pro re nata* – meaning 'according to circumstances' or 'as the situation requires'). A reluctance to give opioids more frequently than this has a major role in the lack of effectiveness of IM regimens. Even if pain returns before the end of this period, which is not uncommon, patients are often made to wait until the 4 hours has elapsed before they are 'allowed' another injection.

Figure 4.1 is a hypothetical representation of what could happen to the blood concentrations of a typical opioid with a half-life of about 3 hours (e.g. morphine or meperidine) if a fixed IM dose is repeated at 4-hourly intervals.

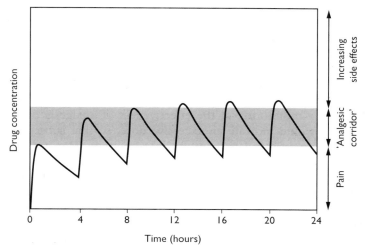

Figure 4.1 Intermittent intramuscular opioid analgesia

analgesia (PCA) after major surgery. Dose requirements may be lower following less major surgery or higher for patients with a history of prior opioid use. Variations may also occur with different patient populations.

Staff are often tempted to start at the lower limit of any prescribed range, but these ranges should allow them the ability to decrease as well as increase subsequent doses as needed. Unless there is a contraindication (e.g. the patient has severe pain or is a little sleepy) and provided the range ordered is appropriate, it is reasonable to start in the middle of the dose range in most cases.

Dose interval

The aims of a dose interval are to allow the previous dose to exert its effect before an additional dose is given and, to a lesser extent, provide an indication of how long a single dose might be expected to have an effect.

PRN dose regimens

Prescriptions of opioids PRN have been the mainstay of acute pain management (albeit often inadequate pain management) for years. There are both drawbacks and advantages to the PRN system. It should mean that opioid is given when the patient needs it. However, there are frequently long delays between the return of discomfort and the actual administration of more opioid. For a variety of reasons a patient may be reluctant to request another injection, at least until pain is severe. In addition, there are the inevitable delays that follow such a request in many hospitals, as opioids are kept in locked cupboards and extra nurses may be required to check the drug and dose before it is given. Following administration there is yet another delay while the drug takes effect. Unless the patient is offered pain relief frequently, or asks for and is given another dose as soon as the pain starts to become uncomfortable, the PRN system will fail.

The main advantage of a PRN regimen is that, titrated properly, it can provide the flexibility needed to cover the changes in pain stimulus that occur within each patient with acute pain.

With a PRN regimen, a dose interval really only has to ensure that a dose of opioid has had its maximum effect before another is given. For an IM injection, this is the time taken for the drug to be absorbed and reach a peak blood concentration plus the time taken to exert its maximum effect on the central nervous system. In most patients this would occur within an hour. Therefore, if a patient is in pain, there is no need to wait 4 hours before giving the next dose. A reasonable dose interval that allows for both safety and flexibility would be 2 hours; some treatment algorithms suggest 1 hour. This does not mean that the drug has to be given every 1 or 2 hours but that it can be given if needed.

Fixed-interval dose regimens

Intramuscular opioids can also be given at fixed intervals. One reason for this approach being less popular than PRN regimens may be that opioid requirements vary enormously between patients and can be difficult to predict. In addition, especially after major injury or operation, the level of pain can fluctuate markedly within each patient according to different pain stimuli (physiotherapy or dressing changes, for example) as well as decrease a little each day. Fixed-interval dosing may not allow adequate flexibility and coverage of these episodes of 'incident' pain or allow for the progressive reduction in dose requirements that will occur as the patient recovers. If fixed-interval regimens are used a range of doses should be available and the interval may need to be less than the traditional 4 hours. Additional PRN opioid orders may also be needed for breakthrough pain.

Monitoring

As outlined in Chapter 2, monitoring of pain scores, sedation scores and respiratory rates will give an indication of 'how much is enough' and 'how much is too much' opioid. For intermittent IM regimens, it would be reasonable to record these values when an injection is given (assuming it is given truly 'on demand') and 1 hour later, when the full effect of the injection can be seen. As with all opioids the aim is to make the patient comfortable while keeping the sedation score less than 2 (see **Box 2.7**).

The onset of other opioid-related side effects, such as nausea and vomiting or pruritus, may be distressing to the patient. If nausea and vomiting appear to be related to the opioid (there are many other causes of postoperative emesis) it may be reasonable to try smaller subsequent doses as well as administer an antiemetic. Individual patients may be more sensitive to one particular opioid, so changing to another opioid is worth considering if other measures have failed.

If the patient complains of pruritus it is worth trying a different opioid. Morphine in particular is associated with a higher incidence of itching than meperidine (pethidine) and fentanyl. As pruritus is not necessarily due to histamine release, antihistamines may not be completely effective and, when administered with opioids, can increase the risk of respiratory depression. Intravenous nalbuphine (2.5–5 mg 4-hourly PRN) may be useful in some cases when other measures have been ineffective.

Selection of subsequent doses

Although the dose range ordered and the initial dose given should be based on the age of the patient, subsequent doses need to be titrated to suit each patient. All too often subsequent doses are chosen because 'that was the dose given before' and not on the basis of patient assessment. A suggested protocol for this titration is outlined in **Box 4.2**. Where possible, patients should be allowed some input into the size and timing of subsequent doses. They can be instructed to ask for a larger subsequent dose if analgesia was inadequate or a smaller dose if they felt sleepy or nauseated.

INTERMITTENT SUBCUTANEOUS ADMINISTRATION

The subcutaneous route is often used for opioid administration in the treatment of cancer pain; it has now become increasingly popular in the management of acute pain.

Box 4.2
Guidelines for intermittent subcutaneous/intramuscular opioid administration. Reproduced with the permission of the Acute Pain Service, Royal Adelaide Hospital

Royal Adelaide Hospital Guidelines

Intermittent Subcutaneous/Intramuscular Opioid Administration For Acute Pain Management

- Pethidine should NOT be given subcutaneously
- For intermittent administration of intravenous opioids refer to appropriate RAH guidelines

Note: Recommended morphine doses are based on average analgesic requirements of patients following major surgery. Consideration should be given to dosage amendment in differing clinical situations

Table: Initial Morphine Orders

Age (Years)	Dose range (mg)
< 15	*
15 – 39	7.5 – 12.5
40 –59	5.0 – 10.0
60 – 69	2.5 – 7.5
70 – 85	2.5 – 5.0
>85	2.0 – 3.0

• Order 2 hourly prn

- Suggest start in middle of dose range
- Upper limit of dose range can be increased if analgesia is inadequate and sedation score is less than 2
- * Contact Drug Information Centre or WCH for advice on opioid doses for children < 15 years

Sedation Score

0	None	
1	Mild	Occasionally drowsy, easy to rouse
2	Moderate	Constantly drowsy, easy to rouse
3	Severe	Somnolent, difficult to rouse
S		Normally asleep

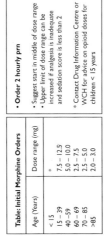

BEGIN

Patient is uncomfortable (in pain) and is offered and/or requests pain relief

Is an opioid ordered? (a valid order is: **2 hourly prn; dose range as in table**)
— No → Get order
— Yes ↓

Record sedation score, respiratory rate and pain score. Is sedation score less than 2 and respiratory rate greater than 8/min?
— No → Seek medical advice
— Yes ↓

Give injection

One hour later record sedation score, respiratory rate and pain score

Is sedation score less than 2 and respiratory rate greater than 8/min?
— No → Seek medical advice. Hold further doses until sedation score less than 2 and respiratory rate greater than 8/min. Consider use of naloxone 100 microgram increments IV.
— Yes ↓

Is patient uncomfortable (in pain) and/or requests another injection?
— No → Reassess later

Is sedation score less than 2 and respiratory rate greater than 8/min?
— No → Seek medical advice. Hold further doses until sedation score less than 2 and respiratory rate greater than 8/min. Consider use of naloxone 100 microgram increments IV.
— Yes ↓

It is more than 2 hours since patient had last dose?
— No → Seek advice about giving injection before 2 hours
— Yes ↓

Repeat same dose unless clinical situation altered

Increase the size of subsequent doses

Decrease the size of subsequent doses

An indwelling narrow-gauge 'butterfly' needle or small IV cannula is inserted into subcutaneous tissue, for ease of access often just below the clavicle or the upper outer aspect of the arm, and covered with a transparent dressing. To ensure that the needle is placed correctly and not too superficially, a generous fold of skin and subcutaneous tissue should be held in one hand and the needle or cannula inserted at the base of this fold (at an angle of 30–45 degrees to the patient) with the other. Injections can be administered through a cap or one-way valve on the indwelling needle. Advantages of using this route over the IM route include improved patient comfort, as the number of skin punctures is decreased, and a reduced risk of needlestick injury – once the indwelling needle is in place, all other needles can be avoided.

If the injection through the indwelling needle is painful it may be that the rate of injection is too rapid (each dose needs to be given over 1–2 minutes) or that the needle has been inserted too superficially. The insertion site should be changed if pain on injection persists or if any redness or swelling develops at the site. Normally the indwelling needle will only need to be replaced every 3–4 days, although some institutions may require all indwelling cannulae to be changed at more frequent intervals.

Morphine is the drug most commonly used for intermittent SC injection. Meperidine (pethidine) tends to be too irritating and painful to be given by this route as a single injection. If meperidine is diluted and given as an infusion or by PCA, irritation is not usually a problem. Subcutaneous opioids should be given in solutions concentrated enough to avoid the need for large volumes as this can be another source of tissue irritation. As the rate of uptake of morphine into the circulation after injection into subcutaneous tissue is similar to the uptake following an IM injection, the dose, dose interval and guidelines for titration are the same as for IM morphine (**Box 4.2**).

ORAL ADMINISTRATION

Delays in gastric emptying are common after surgery and injury. Because of this and the possibility of postoperative nausea and vomiting, the use of oral opioids for the treatment of moderate to severe acute pain has not been common practice. If gastric emptying is delayed the opioids will not pass through to the small intestine where they are absorbed. If several doses are given before normal gastric motility is re-established, they may all enter the small intestine at the same time when emptying resumes. Once a postoperative or post-injury patient is able to tolerate unrestricted amounts of oral fluids, gastric emptying is returning to normal and there is usually no need to continue administration of parenteral opioids.

Commonly, only nonopioid or nonopioid/opioid combination medications are prescribed for oral administration. All too frequently they are the only analgesics ordered to follow PCA or epidural analgesia. They are also often the only analgesia given to patients to take home after day surgery. If the patient has moderate to severe pain these drugs may not provide adequate pain relief.

More potent opioids will be more effective, provided the differences between oral and parenteral doses are understood. Larger doses are required when opioids are given orally compared with doses required for parenteral administration because of the first pass effect: that is, the proportion of an orally administered drug that is metabolized by the liver and/or gut wall after absorption from the gastrointestinal tract determines the amount of unchanged drug that reaches the systemic circulation. The equianalgesic doses of oral and parenteral opioids are listed in **Box 2.2** in Chapter 2.

IMMEDIATE-RELEASE OR CONTROLLED-RELEASE FORMULATIONS

Controlled-release (CR) preparations of morphine (and more recently, oxycodone) are commonly used for the treatment of chronic and cancer pain and usually need to be given only two or three times a day (on a time-contingent basis and not PRN). However, the slower onset (3–4 hours or more to peak effect) and longer duration of action of CR formulations make rapid titration of the drug impossible. The full effect of any dose adjustment may not be seen for a couple of days so these preparations are unsuitable for the treatment of acute pain, at least in the initial stages.

Immediate-release (IR) oral opioids (e.g. oxycodone, morphine syrup, and hydromorphone) are preferred for the early management of acute pain. In most cases analgesia will be obtained within 45–60 minutes, which means that titration to effect will be easier than with CR preparations.

Although methadone has a relatively quick onset of action, its long half-life makes it more difficult to titrate rapidly without risking accumulation of the drug, so it too is unsuitable for the routine management of acute pain.

When patients with chronic or cancer pain are prescribed CR morphine they are often also ordered IR morphine (morphine syrup) for 'breakthrough' analgesia. The amount of IR morphine required can also be used as a guide to altering the dose of CR morphine. The IR morphine can be given when needed (up to 1-hourly PRN if staffing and monitoring permit; often ordered 2–4-hourly PRN) so that the total amount of morphine the patient needs can be rapidly gauged. Immediate-release morphine is usually ordered for breakthrough pain in doses of about one sixth to one tenth of the total daily CR morphine dose.

Example

A 48-year-old patient with metastatic breast cancer has been prescribed 30 mg CR morphine 12-hourly for pain but says that the pain relief is inadequate. She has also been ordered 5–10 mg morphine syrup 2-hourly PRN:

> she required 7 doses of the morphine syrup in 24 hours = 70 mg = 35 mg 12-hourly
> therefore CR morphine could be increased to 60 mg 12-hourly breakthrough doses of morphine syrup could be increased to 15–20 mg

A similar method would be used to assess CR oxycodone doses.

TITRATION OF ORAL OPIOIDS

Titration of oral opioids is very similar to that for IM and SC opioids once allowances are made for equianalgesic doses.

Dose range

As for other routes of opioid administration, doses of oral opioid should be based on the age of the patient. If the patient has been receiving parenteral opioids, particularly via PCA, the parenteral opioid requirement can be used as a guide to the dose of oral opioid that is likely to be needed. If a dose – especially one based on prior parenteral opioid requirements – appears to have no effect, a delay in gastric emptying should be suspected and consideration given to returning to parenteral opioids.

Oxycodone and codeine are two opioids commonly given orally for the treatment of acute pain. Oxycodone is often classed as a 'weak' opioid, but it is not. The amount that can be given orally is only limited by the number of tablets that a patient can reasonably be expected to swallow in one dose (usually no more than eight or ten, i.e. 40–50 mg). If formulations are used where oxycodone is combined with acetaminophen (paracetamol) or aspirin, it is the limits placed on the doses of these drugs that will limit the total amount of oxycodone that can be given in one day. Similarly, oral codeine is commonly administered in a tablet form that combines it with acetaminophen, and therefore the amount of codeine that can be given is limited.

Oral propoxyphene, also usually marketed in a combination formulation, is generally given only for the treatment of mild pain.

Dose interval

As with IM and SC regimens, oral opioids can be ordered as PRN or fixed-interval doses. The onset of action of oral opioids is a little slower than that of intermittent IM/SC injections and a PRN regimen may not be entirely successful, especially if pain is still moderate to severe and the dose required is reasonably large. An alternative is to give the drug at a fixed interval (e.g. strictly 4-hourly) and vary the dose. This interval can be shorter than 4 hours if needed, or medication for breakthrough pain can be ordered in addition to the fixed-interval opioid. Knowledge of a patient's prior opioid requirements (e.g. if a patient is switching from PCA) makes fixed-interval dosing much easier as it gives a good guide to the patient's likely 24-hour oral opioid requirement. Ideally, the patient should be allowed to choose the dose of opioid from the range ordered based on the effect of previous doses.

Monitoring and selection of subsequent doses

Pain scores, sedation scores and respiratory rate should be monitored as for IM/SC opioids.

INTERMITTENT INTRAVENOUS ADMINISTRATION

Many books and guidelines still suggest that IV opioids should be given in doses similar to those administered by IM injection and at similar dose intervals. **Figure 4.2** is a hypothetical representation of what might happen to opioid blood levels if the *same dose* of opioid administered by IM injection in **Figure 4.1** were given by IV injection every 4 hours. This regimen would result in large variations in blood concentrations of the drug, and

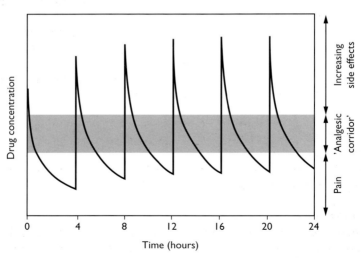

Figure 4.2 Intermittent intravenous opioid analgesia

it is not a particularly effective way of administering opioids. If sustained pain relief is to be obtained without side effects, much smaller doses have to be given much more often. A protocol that has been widely used for the administration of intermittent IV bolus doses of opioid is reproduced in **Box 4.3**. It is managed by nursing staff, usually in the post-anesthesia recovery areas or other specialized areas such as the burns unit. There is no limit to the total amount of opioid that can be given.

The smaller the dose and the more often it can be administered, the less variability there will be in the blood levels of the drug and the easier it will be to titrate the drug to suit each patient and differing pain stimuli. This is the rationale behind PCA and one of the reasons why PCA has been so effective. However, it would be a major logistical and staffing problem if intermittent IV doses of opioid had to be given by nursing staff to large numbers of patients, so this method of analgesia is not recommended for routine maintenance of pain relief in general wards. This technique is, however, the best way to obtain rapid analgesia and should be used to:

- obtain initial pain relief (e.g. immediately after an operation), i.e. 'load' the patient so that blood levels rapidly reach the MEAC for that patient
- provide analgesia for patients who are hypovolemic or hypotensive, when uptake of drug from muscle or subcutaneous tissue is poor
- cover episodes of 'incident pain' (e.g. dressing changes, physiotherapy) or inadequate analgesia

TITRATION OF INTERMITTENT IV OPIOIDS

Dose range

As before, dose ranges should be based on the age of the patient. Suggested doses for morphine are listed in **Box 4.4**.

Dose interval

It may take 15 minutes or more for a less lipid-soluble drug like morphine to exert its maximum effect on the central nervous system after IV administration. However, this interval is too long

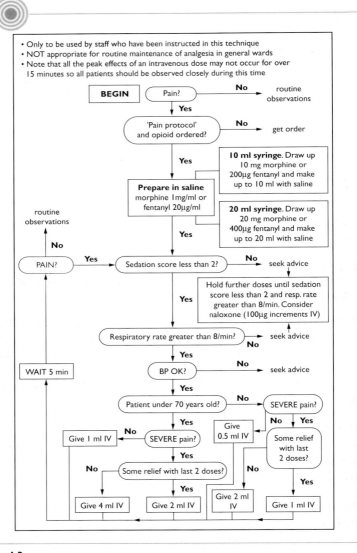

- Only to be used by staff who have been instructed in this technique
- NOT appropriate for routine maintenance of analgesia in general wards
- Note that all the peak effects of an intravenous dose may not occur for over 15 minutes so all patients should be observed closely during this time

BEGIN → Pain? → **No** → routine observations

↓ **Yes**

'Pain protocol' and opioid ordered? → **No** → get order

↓ **Yes**

10 ml syringe. Draw up 10 mg morphine or 200µg fentanyl and make up to 10 ml with saline

Prepare in saline morphine 1mg/ml or fentanyl 20µg/ml

20 ml syringe. Draw up 20 mg morphine or 400µg fentanyl and make up to 20 ml with saline

↓ **Yes**

routine observations

↑ **No**

PAIN? → **Yes** → Sedation score less than 2? → **No** → seek advice

↓ **Yes**

Hold further doses until sedation score less than 2 and resp. rate greater than 8/min. Consider naloxone (100µg increments IV)

↓ **Yes**

Respiratory rate greater than 8/min? → **No** → seek advice

↓ **Yes**

WAIT 5 min

BP OK? → **No** → seek advice

↓ **Yes**

Patient under 70 years old? → **No** → SEVERE pain?

Give 0.5 ml IV

↓ **Yes**

Give 1 ml IV ← **No** ← SEVERE pain?

No | **Yes**

Some relief with last 2 doses?

↓ **Yes**

Some relief with last 2 doses?

No

↓ **Yes**

Give 4 ml IV — Give 2 ml IV — Give 2 ml IV — Give 1 ml IV

Box 4.3

Guidelines for intermittent intravenous opioid administration. Reproduced with permission of the Acute Pain Service, Royal Adelaide Hospital

Titration of intermittent intravenous opioids

Requires:

An age-related range of morphine doses (suggested doses are examples only)	< 70 years: 1 mg, 2 mg or 4 mg > 70 years: 0.5 mg, 1 mg or 2 mg
An appropriate dose interval	3–5 minutes*
Monitoring of pain score, sedation score and respiratory rate	see Box 4.3
Monitoring for presence of other side effects	
Selection of subsequent doses according to patient response	see Box 4.3

Aims for:

Patient comfort, sedation score < 2 and respiratory rate > 8/min

Box 4.4

*The peak effect of the dose will not be seen within 3–5 minutes for all opioids.

if analgesia is to be obtained rapidly. A reasonable balance between absolute safety (ensuring one dose has had its peak effect before another dose is given) and efficacy is to use a dose interval of 3–5 minutes. This has proved safe and effective, as long as staff monitor the patient carefully and are aware that this interval may not represent the true time to peak effect.

Monitoring and selection of subsequent doses

A protocol is given in **Box 4.3**. While this protocol is in use and for 15 minutes after cessation of the protocol, a nurse should remain close to the patient.

Subsequent analgesic regimens

Patients given intermittent IV opioids will normally be changed to an alternative analgesic regimen once comfortable. If PCA is to be used it can be started immediately. If IM or SC opioids are ordered a dose should be given at the earliest sign of discomfort.

CONTINUOUS INTRAVENOUS INFUSIONS

In an attempt to avoid the 'peaks and troughs' in blood concentration associated with intermittent administration, continuous intravenous infusions of opioid are sometimes used in the management of acute pain. While it may be possible to maintain reasonably constant blood levels using this technique, it is difficult to predict what the level will need to be for a particular patient or what dose is needed to achieve it. Also, acute pain is not constant and the amount of opioid required by a patient will vary in response to different pain stimuli. For the reasons outlined below, alterations of infusion rate alone will often mean there is a considerable delay in matching the amount of opioid delivered to the amount of opioid actually needed. There are also possible risks from blood levels of the drug that may continue to rise after analgesia has been obtained.

If an infusion of any drug is ordered at a fixed rate, it takes five half-lives of the drug to reach 95% of final steady state concentration. The half-life of morphine is 2–3 hours, so it may take up to 15 hours for blood levels to reach a plateau at this steady state concentration. It is this plateau that needs to be in the 'analgesic corridor'.

It can be seen from the hypothetical representation in **Figure 4.3** of a continuous infusion of an opioid with a half-life of 3 hours (e.g. morphine or meperidine) that analgesia has been obtained within 3 hours of starting the infusion. If this infusion continues at the same rate, the blood concentration will continue to rise for some hours, and side effects (including respiratory depression) may result. It will also take hours for each alteration made to the infusion rate to have its full effect, i.e. to reach the new steady state concentration – a fact often not recognized by staff who may change the rates as often as every 30 minutes.

A patient who becomes sedated while using PCA (PCA mode only) will not press the demand button and further doses of opioid will not be delivered. Equipment used for continuous infusions of opioid will continue to deliver the drug regardless of whether the patient is sedated or not. For this reason continuous

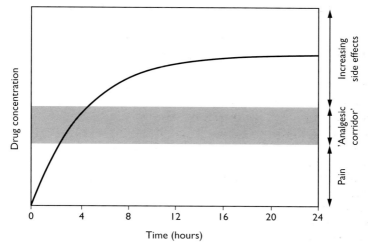

Figure 4.3 Continuous intravenous opioid infusions

intravenous opioid infusions are probably the *least safe* way to administer opioids in a general ward.

TITRATION OF CONTINUOUS IV OPIOID INFUSIONS
Dose range

In view of the variable time taken from the commencement of a continuous infusion to the onset of pain relief, analgesia will be obtained more rapidly if IV bolus doses (as in **Box 4.4**) are administered to 'load' the patient in the first instance, and the infusion commenced once the patient is comfortable. It has been said that the rate of the infusion can then be based on this loading dose – half the loading dose being required during each elimination half-life. However, half-lives vary between patients; various opioid doses may have been given during surgery; pain immediately after surgery may differ from pain later in the ward (e.g. shoulder tip pain after laparoscopy or abdominal colic may have abated); sedation after anesthesia may have limited the amount of opioid given; and the volume status of the patient may have altered (hypovolemia reducing the amount of opioid needed). These and other variables make this calculation, at best, a guide.

Monitoring

Sedation scores, pain scores and respiratory rates should be monitored frequently, and hourly intervals are suggested.

Alterations of infusion rates

Because of the time taken for any alteration in infusion rate to have an effect, if analgesia is inadequate, IV bolus doses should again be used to achieve patient comfort before the infusion rate is increased.

If an infusion is stopped it also take five half-lives of the drug to return to a blood concentration of zero. Therefore if a patient becomes oversedated, the infusion should cease until the patient is more awake (sedation score less than 2), not merely be reduced to a lower rate.

RECTAL ADMINISTRATION

The submucosal venous plexus of the rectum drains into the superior, middle and inferior rectal veins. Drug absorbed from the lower half of the rectum will pass into the latter two veins and into the inferior vena cava, thus bypassing the portal vein and first-pass metabolism in the liver. This is one of the advantages of this route of administration. Drug absorbed through the rectal mucosa of the upper part of the rectum passes into the superior rectal vein and enters the portal system.

Rectal absorption is often variable owing to differences in the site of placement of the drug, the contents of the rectum and the blood supply to the rectum. In addition, there is not always widespread patient – or indeed staff – acceptance of this route of administration. The drug may not be distributed evenly throughout the suppository and therefore doses of 'half a suppository' may not deliver half of the amount of opioid in that suppository.

CHAPTER 5

PATIENT-CONTROLLED ANALGESIA

Equipment

Contraindications

Programmable variables

Standard orders and nursing procedure protocols

Subsequent analgesic regimens

Complications

Alternative routes

Patient-controlled analgesia (PCA), in a broad sense, is not restricted to a single route or method of analgesic administration or a single class of analgesic drug, but means that patients can determine when and how much analgesic they receive. However, the term is more commonly used to describe a method of pain relief which employs sophisticated infusion devices and allows patients to self-administer opioids, usually intravenously.

Generally, in hospital wards, PCA has been associated with better pain relief and greater patient satisfaction compared with intermittent opioid injections. The reasons for this include:

- small and frequent intravenous bolus doses of opioid can be given whenever the patient becomes uncomfortable, enabling individual titration of pain relief and maintenance of blood concentrations of opioid within their therapeutic range (analgesic corridor) (**Figure 5.1**).
- this flexibility helps to overcome the wide interpatient variation in opioid requirements (eightfold to tenfold) in each age group (see Chapter 2)
- the intensity of acute pain is rarely constant and PCA means that the amount of opioid delivered can be rapidly

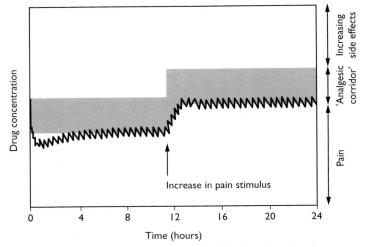

Figure 5.1 Patient-controlled analgesia is more likely to keep blood concentrations of opioid within the 'analgesic corridor' and allows rapid titration if there is an increase in pain stimulus, requiring higher blood levels of opioid in order to maintain analgesia

titrated if pain increases and higher blood levels of drug are required before analgesia is once again obtained

- patients are able to titrate the amount of opioid delivered against dose-related side effects

Many institutions have only a few PCA machines. Patients who benefit from PCA most are those who have had major surgery and are not permitted oral fluids (and who therefore cannot take oral analgesics), those with marked 'incident' pain (e.g. associated with fractured ribs, physiotherapy or dressing changes), and those who cannot be given intramuscular injections even for a short time (e.g. hemophiliac patients or patients on anticoagulants).

This chapter focuses on the use of opioids with PCA. Much less often, admixtures of an opioid with another drug (such as ketamine) are used. However, large interpatient variations in postoperative opioid requirements mean that patients are likely to receive widely varying doses of the added drug. This could lead to inadequate therapy in some patients and an increased risk of adverse effects in others.

EQUIPMENT

There are two types of PCA device:
- microprocessor-controlled syringe pumps
- disposable devices

MICROPROCESSOR-CONTROLLED SYRINGE PUMPS

Microprocessor-controlled syringe pumps deliver, within preset limits, a bolus dose of drug when the patient presses a demand button connected to the pump. Access to the syringe (or other drug reservoir) and the microprocessor program are only possible using a key or an access code. Certain variables are prescribed and programmed into the PCA machine (see below) and control how much opioid the patient can receive. Most machines can also deliver a continuous or background infusion, thus PCA machines can operate in three modes:
- PCA mode only
- continuous infusion only
- a combination of PCA with a continuous (background) infusion

Patients using PCA (PCA mode) are instructed to push the demand button whenever they are uncomfortable. If the PCA machine has a pneumatic demand mechanism and the patient is unable to use either hand, a piece of plastic tubing can be attached to the machine instead of the hand-held button and the patient instructed to blow into this tubing. Some machines will also operate with a pressure-sensitive pad or foot pedal.

The inherent safety of the technique lies in the fact that, as long as the machine is in PCA mode only (i.e. there is no continuous infusion), further doses of opioid will not be delivered should the patient become excessively sedated, because no further demands will be made. This assumes that the patient is the only one pressing the button. Staff must explain to the patient, relatives and friends that no one but the patient is allowed to operate the PCA machine.

DISPOSABLE PCA DEVICES

A number of disposable PCA devices have been developed. These deliver a fixed volume of drug following each demand. One of the disadvantages of a fixed-volume system is that the concentration of drug in the reservoir must be changed if increases or decreases in the size of the incremental bolus dose are required. In addition, the drug reservoir is easily accessible and the security of controlled drugs may be compromised in the hospital setting.

CONTRAINDICATIONS

The contraindications to PCA are summarized in **Box 5.1**. A current or past history of addiction to opioid drugs was often thought to be a contraindication. It is now realized that PCA can be a useful way of managing acute pain in this population, when supervised by pain medicine specialists. Much larger opioid doses than usual will often be required.

UNTRAINED NURSING AND MEDICAL STAFF

Patient-controlled analgesia is an effective way of providing good pain relief, but results depend on a good understanding of the technique. Therefore, PCA should only be used by medical and nursing staff who have the appropriate training. An inadequate

Contraindications to PCA

- untrained staff (nursing and medical)
- patient rejection
- patient inability to comprehend the technique (e.g. language barrier, confusion)
- extremes of age

Box 5.1

understanding of PCA, the drugs and doses used, the monitoring requirements and the management of common problems can, at worst, increase the risk of complications. At best, it can prove to be a very expensive way of providing suboptimal analgesia.

Nursing education and accreditation programs that have to be completed by each nurse before he or she can take responsibility for a patient with PCA are recommended. If this is done, nursing staff may be able to program PCA machines, change syringes and make alterations to the program according to the PCA standard orders.

In many institutions the use of PCA is supervised by anesthesiologists.

PATIENT REJECTION

The majority of patients appreciate the control that PCA gives them and the ability to rapidly titrate their own analgesia and balance pain relief with the degree of any side effects that may occur. This is one of the reasons that patients using PCA sometimes express a greater satisfaction with this technique compared with others such as epidural analgesia, even though the degree of pain relief may be less. Patients' wish for control, their locus of control (see Chapter 12), and their level of self-efficacy may all influence their use of PCA. Some patients may not want this control and would prefer the nursing and medical staff to manage their pain relief.

INABILITY TO COMPREHEND THE TECHNIQUE

For PCA to be used both safely and effectively the patient must be able to understand the technique. Patients should not automatically be excluded from consideration if there is mild mental impairment or a language barrier. Relatives or translators can be asked to interpret verbal instructions about the use of PCA, and patient education leaflets can be written in many languages. However, if staff feel that despite these measures the patient still does not understand PCA, alternative methods of pain relief will be needed. Patients who are confused will often not be offered PCA and those who become confused may need to have PCA discontinued.

An understanding of PCA does not necessarily have to be detailed. Some elderly patients have thought that the hand-held button contained a 'magic beam' and needed to be directed at the site of pain before being pressed (problems only arise if they attempt to treat other patients' pain as well!). Other patients have used the button as they would a bronchodilator inhaler, that is, when they require another dose they bring the button to their mouth, press it and inhale. As long as they are aware that the button is pressed only when they become uncomfortable, the patient may be allowed to continue with PCA.

PATIENT AGE

The technique has been used successfully in patients of almost all ages. Many children as young as 4 years old, as well as patients in their 90s, can manage PCA very well as long as they understand the explanations given and are willing to be active participants in their own care.

PROGRAMMABLE VARIABLES

There are many different models of microprocessor-controlled PCA machine now available. Although the variables that can be programmed into the machines differ a little, a number of features are common to most of them. Commonly used settings for PCA variables are listed in **Box 5.2**.

LOADING DOSE

Patient-controlled analgesia is a maintenance therapy. That is, it is a good way to maintain patient comfort but an ineffective way of achieving that comfort in the first place. It may not be effective if moderate or severe pain is present at commencement. To make the patient comfortable before PCA is started, a loading dose of opioid is needed. There is an enormous interpatient variation in the amount of opioid required as a loading dose and it may be better to individualize this dose for each patient (e.g. by using the protocols in Chapter 4) rather than program a single loading dose via the PCA machine.

Commonly prescribed initial values for PCA variables in opioid-naive patients

Variable	Value	Comments
Loading dose	0 mg (i.e. zero)	• best to titrate for each patient before starting PCA
Incremental dose (bolus dose)	morphine 1 mg meperidine 10 mg diamorphine 0.5 mg fentanyl 20 µg hydromorphone 0.2 mg tramadol 10 mg	• consider starting with doses half these amounts in patients over 70 years old • the dose may need to be increased if analgesia is inadequate
Concentration	variable	• best if standardized for each drug
Dose duration	cannot be adjusted in most PCA machines but where this can be done 'stat' is the shortest dose duration	
Lock-out period	5 min to 8 min	
Background infusion	0 mg/h (i.e. zero)	• see text for exceptions • if used, the rate of infusion in mg/h is usually no greater than the bolus dose in mg
1-h or 4-h limits	30 mg morphine (or equivalent) in 4 h	• consider varying according to patient age • consider omitting

Box 5.2

After regional anesthesia, moderate to severe pain can occur rapidly as the local anesthetic block wears off. The use of PCA alone may be ineffective in controlling this pain and a method to load the patient must be available, even if the patient has returned to the ward after surgery.

INCREMENTAL (BOLUS) DOSE

The bolus dose is the amount of opioid (in milligrams or micrograms) that the PCA machine will deliver when the demand button is pressed. Many opioids have been used with PCA (morphine being the most common) but those having very short or very long durations of action are not usually recommended. Partial agonist or agonist-antagonist opioids are used far less commonly than pure opioid agonists.

The size of the incremental dose, along with the lock-out interval (see below), can determine the effectiveness of PCA. If the dose is too small patients will not be able to obtain adequate analgesia; if the dose is too large there may be an unacceptable incidence of side effects. Commonly used initial dose sizes (in opioid-naive patients) are given in **Box 5.2**. The optimal incremental dose for each patient is one that consistently results in appreciable analgesia without side effects. Therefore, adjustments to the size of the initial dose may be required.

With conventional intermittent opioid regimens, the dose of opioid prescribed should be reduced as the age of the patient increases. As patients with PCA can vary the total daily dose according to the number of demands they make, a progressive decrease in dose with increasing age is not necessary. However, patients over 70 years old have, on average, less than half the total daily opioid requirement of a 20-year-old. Therefore it is reasonable to start with smaller PCA incremental doses.

DOSE DURATION

The rate at which the PCA machine delivers the bolus dose can be altered in some machines, allowing the bolus dose to be delivered as an infusion (e.g. over 5 minutes). If subcutaneous PCA is used (see later), rapid delivery of a dose may cause some stinging; a slower rate of delivery will reduce the chance of this occurring.

LOCK-OUT INTERVAL

The time from the *end* of the delivery of one dose until the machine will respond to another demand is called the lock-out interval. This is designed to increase the safety of PCA by allowing the patient to feel the effect of one dose before receiving a subsequent dose. Practically, however, lock-out intervals of 5–8 minutes are commonly prescribed. This is usually the case regardless of the opioid used, even though it may take up to 15 minutes or longer for the peak effect of an IV dose of morphine (most commonly used in PCA) to be seen. A longer lock-out interval reduces the ability of the patient to rapidly titrate the amount of opioid required and therefore decreases the effectiveness of PCA.

When patients are told about the lock-out interval, it is important to ensure that they realize it only means that another dose *can* be delivered, should they press the button, and not that they *need* to press every 5–8 minutes.

Lock-out intervals of 5–8 minutes mean that, allowing for time for the dose to be delivered, a patient could demand and receive up to ten doses of opioid each hour. In reality, if patients feel that a particular incremental dose is not effective, they will not continue to press the demand button. Most patients have an inherent maximum frequency of demand, and it is uncommon for a patient to sustain a demand rate of more than three or four doses per hour. If, despite an average of three or four doses each hour, analgesia is inadequate, it may be preferable to increase the size of the bolus dose rather than decrease the lock-out interval or instruct the patient to press the button more often.

CONTINUOUS (BACKGROUND) INFUSION

Most PCA machines can deliver a continuous infusion. When used at a low rate in addition to PCA mode (patient demand mode), it was hoped that a constant but subanalgesic blood concentration could be maintained. Therefore, when a bolus dose of opioid was delivered, the blood level would reach the analgesic corridor more rapidly. It was also hoped that a continuous infusion would enable the patient to make fewer demands, sleep for longer periods and wake in less pain.

Unfortunately, there is no consistent evidence to suggest that the routine addition of a continuous infusion has the beneficial effects that were anticipated for the average patient. A continuous infusion:

- does not always reduce the number of demands made by the patient
- may increase the total amount of opioid delivered
- has been shown to increase the risk of side effects, including respiratory depression

- does not always result in better analgesia
- does not always result in improved sleep patterns

A continuous infusion reduces the inherent safety of the PCA technique, as opioid will be delivered regardless of the sedation level of the patient.

While the routine use of a background infusion is not recommended, it may be required in some opioid-naive patients and, more commonly, in those who are opioid-tolerant.

Opioid-naive patients

There may be some benefit from the use of a continuous infusion in patients who have high opioid requirements or who complain of waking repeatedly in severe pain at night. In both these situations the daytime opioid requirement of the patient is known and the rate of infusion can be adjusted accordingly. A typical approach is to order a continuous infusion that provides about 50% of a patient's *known* hourly opioid dose. For example, if a patient using 100 mg/day of morphine (2 mg bolus dose) complains of waking in severe pain at night, an infusion rate of 50 mg/day (= 2 mg/hour) could be added. If the combination of a continuous infusion and PCA mode is prescribed in opioid-naive patients, it is recommended that the rate in milligrams per hour should usually not exceed the size of the bolus dose in milligrams.

In acute pain management, daily opioid requirements often decrease rapidly; therefore the need for the infusion, as well as the rate of infusion prescribed, should be reassessed frequently.

Opioid-tolerant patients

In patients who are opioid-tolerant, background infusions may sometimes be used in place of the patient's normal (preadmission) opioid requirements (see Chapter 9).

CONCENTRATION

For consistency and safety, each institution should standardize the concentrations of drugs administered by PCA where possible. Most companies that manufacture PCA machines suggest that the volume delivered following each demand should not be less than 0.5 ml.

HOURLY LIMITS

Hourly or 4-hourly limits prevent the patient receiving more than a designated amount of opioid within a set time. However, large interpatient variations in opioid requirements make it impossible to predict the 'safe' limit for each patient. For example, a commonly prescribed limit is 30 mg of morphine (or equianalgesic doses of an alternative opioid) in 4 hours. This may be inadequate for some patients, yet may be all that an older patient requires in 24 hours.

For PCA to be used effectively, a wide range of opioid requirements needs to be recognized and tolerated. The setting of a dose limit may not mean added safety for patients with low opioid requirements and may prevent those needing higher doses from obtaining good pain relief. Hourly or 4-hourly limits are not present on all machines.

The amount of opioid a patient is 'allowed' should not be influenced by preconceived ideas of maximum doses. In general, patients have not received an excessive dose if they remain unsedated. An exception to this is the use of meperidine (pethidine), when high doses may lead to normeperidine toxicity. As a number of opioids are suitable for use with PCA, it would seem reasonable to restrict the use of meperidine to situations where these other opioids are unavailable.

The setting of a limit could give staff a false sense of security, as they may believe that the patient cannot receive an excessive dose of drug. As with other features designed to increase patient safety with PCA, the setting of a dose limit cannot compensate for any shortcomings in monitoring.

STANDARD ORDERS AND NURSING PROCEDURE PROTOCOLS

To maximize the effectiveness of PCA and minimize the risk of complications, standard orders and nursing procedure protocols are recommended. However, even when these are used, PCA may be more effective when supervised by an acute pain service team compared with less experienced medical staff.

STANDARD ORDERS

To standardize orders throughout the institution, preprinted forms are suggested. The forms need to be completed, signed and dated by the treating doctor. Examples of preprinted pain management flow sheets and PCA standard order forms are given at the end of this chapter.

Standard orders can be a safe and effective way of initiating treatment with PCA. However, the orders may not be suitable for all patients. Daily evaluation (or more often if required) will allow appropriate alterations to be made so that maximum therapeutic benefit can be obtained with minimum possible side effects. Daily assessment should usually include:

- effectiveness of analgesia at rest and with activity
- effectiveness of the treatment of any side effects
- an overall assessment of the patient, including the possibility of non-PCA-related complications and any concurrent medication orders

Standard orders need to cover the following areas:

Nondrug treatment orders

Nondrug treatment orders may include a statement to eliminate the concurrent ordering of CNS depressants or other opioids by others; orders for oxygen; the need for a one-way 'antireflux' valve to be sited in the IV line (to prevent the opioid traveling back up the primary IV line should the IV cannula become obstructed); and instructions as to whom to contact if problems occur.

Monitoring and documentation requirements

As with any opioid regimen used for the management of acute pain, the pain score, sedation score and respiratory rate should be monitored. These should be recorded at regular intervals, along with the total amount of opioid delivered, the dose of any drug administered for the treatment of side effects, and any changes that have been made to the PCA program.

The monitoring and recording of these parameters allows a regular assessment of the progress of each patient and for rational changes to be made to PCA orders so that treatment is individualized. It should be noted that most patients will titrate their pain relief to a level at which they are comfortable and not aim for complete analgesia, even in the absence of opioid-related side effects.

Certain higher-risk patients, such as the morbidly obese and those with sleep apnea or severe pulmonary disease, will require additional and closer observation during the first 24 hours using PCA. Continuous pulse oximetry should be considered.

PCA orders

All variables of the PCA program need to be prescribed (see **Box 5.2**). As well, it is helpful to have orders that enable staff to increase or decrease the size of the bolus dose (within set limits) if needed.

Orders for the treatment of side effects

The inclusion of standard orders for the recognition and management of opioid-related side effects will minimize delays in treatment.

Nursing procedure protocols

The format of nursing procedure protocols for PCA will vary with each institution, but there are elements that need to be included in each, regardless of format. These are listed in **Box 5.3**.

SUBSEQUENT ANALGESIC REGIMENS

Opioid requirements during PCA can be used as guide for the opioid regimen to be used once PCA has been discontinued. If the patient is tolerating unlimited oral fluids, oral opioids can be ordered. If PCA must cease before oral fluids can be given, other parenteral (intramuscular, subcutaneous or intravenous) opioids will be needed. In general, PCA is maintained until oral opioids can be used.

There should be some overlap of pain therapies so that the subsequent regimen has time to have an effect before PCA is stopped. If there is to be a change in clinician responsibility for

Elements of intravenous PCA nursing procedure protocols

- a statement of the institution policy towards accreditation for nursing staff responsible for a patient with PCA
- a statement indicating who has responsibility for writing PCA orders
- a guide to the location of keys for PCA machines (usually with Controlled Substances keys)
- mechanisms for the checking and discarding of PCA opioids
- guidelines for the suitability, or otherwise, of patients for PCA
- instructions and guidelines for preoperative patient education
- monitoring and documentation requirements
- availability and use of drugs to treat side effects
- instructions for the checking of the PCA settings against the prescription (e.g. at each shift change and change of syringe)
- instructions for checking the amount of drug delivered (from the machine display) against the amount remaining in the syringe
- detailed instruction on the setting up and programming of the PCA machine
- the use of a one-way antireflux valve
- management of equipment faults and alarms
- instructions about whom to call if assistance or advice is required

Box 5.3

the pain management of the patient, then this change needs to be clearly understood by all staff.

ORAL OPIOIDS

Any of the oral opioids suitable for the management of acute pain may be used following PCA (see Chapter 4). The oral dosage can be based on the amount of IV opioid used in the 24 hours prior to stopping PCA and the equianalgesic doses of PCA and oral opioids (Chapter 2).

As intensity of acute pain usually decreases daily, it is likely that the patient will require less opioid than would be expected based solely on equianalgesic doses (see Chapter 2). The oral regimen therefore needs to accommodate this expected decrease in dose requirement. For example, if oral oxycodone is prescribed to follow IV morphine PCA, the daily oxycodone requirement is likely to be less (based on the equianalgesic doses of 10 mg IV morphine = 20 mg oral oxycodone) than the previous 24-hour PCA morphine requirement. To enable patients to titrate their own analgesia, it may be appropriate to allow the daily oxycodone dose to range between 0.5 and 2 times the last 24-hour PCA morphine requirement. The estimated 24-hour oxycodone dose can then be ordered in six divided doses. As an example:

immediate last 24-hour PCA morphine = 60 mg

therefore,

   next 24-hour oxycodone requirement = 60 mg
   approximately   = 10 mg 4-hourly

therefore

   order a range based on this calculation = 5–20 mg 4-hourly

Depending on clinical circumstances the oral opioid may be ordered on a PRN or time-contingent basis and doses can be given more often than 4-hourly. The 'PCA principle' should continue and patients should, in most cases, have some input into the dose given and the timing of that dose.

If PCA morphine requirements are less than about 30 mg per day, less potent opioid formulations, e.g. a combination of acetaminophen (paracetamol) plus codeine, may suffice. Other analgesics, such as nonsteroidal anti-inflammatory drugs (including acetaminophen), may also be used.

INTRAMUSCULAR OR SUBCUTANEOUS OPIOIDS

To convert PCA morphine requirements to an intermittent intramuscular (IM) or subcutaneous (SC), regimen, the 24-hour PCA dose can be divided by 8 to find the center of an appropriate dose range. As an example:

immediate last 24-hour PCA morphine   = 60 mg

therefore, middle of dose range for IM/SC   = 60 mg ÷ 8
                                       = 7.5 mg

therefore, order a range based on this calculation = 5–10 mg
                                          2-hourly PRN

Although division by 8 estimates a 3-hourly dose, it is reasonable to add additional flexibility by ordering the range of doses 2-hourly PRN (see Chapter 4).

COMPLICATIONS

Complications of PCA may be related to the equipment, the side effects of the opioids or inadequate analgesia.

PROBLEMS RELATED TO THE EQUIPMENT

Equipment malfunction

Interference from current surges or static electricity has led to PCA machine malfunction. Usually this will be 'fail-safe' – for example, the program will default to the lowest setting possible for a bolus dose. However, cases have been recorded where machine malfunction has led to the continuous delivery of the contents of a syringe. Although the risk of this problem is less in later-model machines, it may be wise to check the PCA program whenever the syringe is changed and whenever the machine is connected to or disconnected from mains power. Most machines have a battery back-up that will enable the machine to run for up to 8 hours in the event of a power failure.

Other equipment problems have included cracked syringe barrels, which have allowed the contents of the PCA syringe to empty by gravity, and faulty one-way valves. The PCA machine (and other infusion devices) should be placed at an appropriate level relative to the patient.

Operator error

Operator error can lead to misprogramming of the PCA machine, improper loading of the syringe or incorrect placement of the one-way antireflux valve. Failure to clamp the intravenous (IV) tubing during a syringe change may allow delivery of an inadvertent bolus dose of opioid. Errors in PCA prescriptions have also occurred – either inadvertently or due to an inadequate knowledge of PCA.

Inappropriate patient or nonpatient use

Respiratory depression may occur if the patient does not adequately comprehend the technique. Examples include pushing the demand button every time the lock-out interval ends, or mistaking the button for a nurse-call button. It has also been reported following activation of PCA by well-meaning relatives or friends of the patient, and hospital staff.

Tampering

Despite locked covers on PCA machines, some patients have managed to extract the syringe from some machines without damaging the equipment.

SIDE EFFECTS RELATED TO THE OPIOID

Opioid-related side effects may develop regardless of the route of administration of the drug (see Chapter 2). Outlined in **Box 5.4** are suggested management options should adverse effects occur during the use of PCA. Most opioids have been given via PCA; most studies have failed to show significant differences between them, either in terms of side effects or efficacy.

Nausea and vomiting

If nausea or vomiting occurs, an appropriate antiemetic should be given or, if that antiemetic appears to be ineffective, an alternative ordered. If a patient has low opioid requirements, a decrease in the size of the bolus dose can also be tried. Patients who complain of a wave of nausea or dizziness a few minutes after pressing the demand button may benefit from a smaller bolus dose or a slower rate of infusion of the bolus dose (i.e. an increase in the 'dose duration').

Although there is little evidence to support a difference in the incidence of nausea and vomiting with different opioids, individual patients may appear to be more sensitive to one particular drug. In this case, and if other measures have failed, a change to another opioid is worth considering. It may also be that the opioid is not the cause, or the sole cause, of the nausea and vomiting (see Chapter 2).

Management of inadequate analgesia and side effects of PCA opioids*

Nausea and vomiting
- administer antiemetics (change if ineffective)
- decrease the size of the bolus dose if opioid requirements are low
- increase the dose duration if possible
- consider other possible causes
- change to another opioid
- lie patient flat and minimize movement until treatment has had time to work
- consider transdermal scopolamine (hyoscine) if patient < 60 years old

Pruritus
- check whether it appears to be related to the opioid
- change to another opioid
- ? administer an antihistamine (watch for sedation)
- ? administer naloxone (may reverse analgesia)
- ? nalbuphine

Sedation and respiratory depression
- sedation score 2, respiratory rate > 8/min: reduce (e.g. halve) size of bolus dose
- score 2, respiratory rate < 8/min: reduce size of bolus dose, consider naloxone (100 μg)
- sedation score 3 (regardless of respiratory rate): administer naloxone (100 μg, repeat PRN)

Urinary retention
- catheterize – 'in-out' or indwelling

Confusion
- may not be related to the opioid but PCA may need to cease and alternative analgesia be provided

Normeperidine (norpethidine) toxicity
- prevention is preferred (avoid the use of meperidine or limit total doses given)

Decreased bowel motility
- anticipatory treatment where possible; discourage use of PCA to cover discomfort resulting from resumption of peristalsis

Hypotension
- look for causes of hypovolemia

Box 5.4
  *These strategies are suggestions only and may not be needed in, or suitable for, the treatment of all patients.

As the emetic effects of opioids are enhanced by vestibular stimulation, the patient may feel better lying flat and minimizing movement until any treatment has had time to have an effect. Transdermal scopolamine (hyoscine) is often beneficial in this situation but may be best avoided in patients over 60 years old (although the use of half a patch may be considered).

Pruritus

As outlined in Chapter 2, pruritus may be due to histamine release or a consequence of possible μ receptor activation. It is more common following morphine than meperidine or fentanyl.

After checking that any pruritus is likely to be due to the opioid (i.e. its distribution is over the face and trunk) and if the patient is disturbed by this side effect, the safest treatment in the first instance is to change to another opioid. Antihistamines, because of their sedative effects, may add to the risk of sedation and respiratory depression. Pruritus may also respond to small, carefully titrated doses of intravenous naloxone, but there is a risk that it may reverse the analgesia. Nalbuphine in small IV doses is sometimes effective.

Sedation and respiratory depression

The best clinical indicator of early respiratory depression is sedation. If a patient has a sedation score of 2 (see Chapter 2) a reduction in the size of the PCA bolus dose (e.g. by 50%) is usually indicated. Even if sedatives have been given this may still be the safest course of action – the dose can always be increased again if analgesia is inadequate, once the patient is more alert.

If the patient has a sedation score of 2 and a respiratory rate below 8 breaths per minute, the administration of a small dose of naloxone (100 μg IV) may also be considered in addition to a reduction in the size of the bolus dose. Whether or not naloxone is considered necessary in this instance may depend on factors such as staffing levels. If no nurse is available to keep a continued close watch on the patient, it may be safer to give naloxone. If a patient develops severe respiratory depression with a sedation score of 3 (unrousable), naloxone should be given regardless of the respiratory rate. Remember that naloxone has a shorter half-life than commonly used opioid agonists and repeated doses or an infusion may be needed.

Respiratory depression during PCA therapy has been reported in patients following postoperative hemorrhage. A normally appropriate incremental dose of opioid may become excessive in the presence of hypovolemia. Until the patient is normovolemic, smaller incremental bolus doses may be needed.

Urinary retention

Urinary retention may occur as a result of opioid administration. Whatever the cause, the patient may need to be catheterized – either an 'in-out' or an indwelling catheter.

Confusion

Opioids will not usually be the cause, or the sole cause, of confusion. However, PCA may need to be discontinued as the patient may press the demand button inappropriately. Alternative methods of pain relief should then be organized.

Normeperidine (norpethidine) toxicity

As described in Chapter 2, normeperidine toxicity can follow the administration of large doses of meperidine (pethidine). This is probably more likely following PCA than conventional opioid delivery techniques as PCA has allowed many patients to receive more opioid than they would have done with nurse-administered analgesic regimens in the past.

As many opioids can be used with PCA, it would seem reasonable to restrict the use of meperidine to situations where other drugs are not available. If meperidine must be ordered, it is recommended that the total dose be kept to less than 1000 mg in the first 24 hours of therapy and less than 600–700 mg per day thereafter in the younger patient (and even less in the older patient or those with renal impairment).

Inhibition of bowel motility

To a greater or lesser extent inhibition of bowel motility is an inevitable consequence of the use of opioids. Where possible and if opioids are to be used for some days, treatment should be

Thomas V., Heath M., Rose D. and Flory P. (1995) Psychological characteristics and the effectiveness of patient-controlled analgesia. *British Journal of Anaesthesia* **74**, 271–276.

Woodhouse A., Hobbes A.F.T., Mather L.E. and Gibson M. (1996) A comparison of morphine, pethidine and fentanyl in the postsurgical patient-controlled environment. *Pain* **64**, 115–121.

Woodhouse A., Ward M.E. and Mather L.E. (1999) Intra-subject variability in postoperative patient-controlled analgesia (PCA): is the patient equally satisfied with morphine, pethidine and fentanyl? *Pain* **80**, 545–553.

APPENDIX TO CHAPTER 5

Examples of acute pain management flowsheets and standard orders for patient-controlled analgesia, reproduced with permission of the Acute Pain Services at the Royal Adelaide Hospital, Adelaide, Australia and the University of Washington Medical Center, Seattle, Washington, USA.

5A Royal Adelaide Hospital chart for observations and record of drug administration

5B University of Washington Medical Center pain management flowsheet

5C University of Washington Medical Center intravenous PCA physician order sheet

5D Royal Adelaide Hospital Acute Pain Service PCA standard orders

APPENDIX 5A

ROYAL ADELAIDE HOSPITAL

ACUTE PAIN SERVICE
SPECIAL OBSERVATIONS
AND RECORD OF DRUG
ADMINISTRATION

Unit Record No.: _____

Surname: _____

Given Names: _____

Date of Birth: _____ Sex: _____

Date/Time	Drug	Dose	Pain score .... X 0 2 4 6 8 10	Sed'n	Resp	PR	BP	Comments	Signature MO or RN

APPENDIX 5A

ADVERSE DRUG REACTIONS

Drug	Date	Details	Signature

PAIN SCORE: 0 = no pain   10 = worst pain imaginable

SEDATION SCORE:
0 = none
1 = mild, occasionally drowsy, easy to rouse
2 = moderate, constantly drowsy, easy to rouse
3 = severe, somnolent, difficult to rouse
S = normally asleep, easy to rouse

Date/ Time	Drug	Dose	Pain score .... X 0 2 4 6 8 10	Sed'n	Resp	PR	BP	Comments	Signature MO or RN

APPENDIX 5B

SEDATION SCALE
0 = None
1 = Mild
    (occasionally drowsy; easy to arouse)
2 = Moderate
    (frequently drowsy; easy to arouse)
3 = Severe
    (somnolent; difficult to arouse)
S = Normal sleep
    (easy to arouse)

ANALGESIA SCALE
0 = no pain
10 = worst pain imaginable

MONITORING
PCA: Q ____ hr x ____ hrs;
    then Q ____ hrs

EPIDURAL:
    Q ____ hr x ____ hrs;
    then Q ____ hrs

Date													
Time													
Resp. Rate													
Sedation													
Analgesia													

PATIENT CONTROLLED ANALGESIA

Med (mg/ml)													
Incremental Dose													
Lockout Interval													
4 Hour Limit													
Bolus Dose													
Continuous Infusion													
Cumulative Dose													
Clear volume													
Syringe added													

UNIVERSITY OF WASHINGTON MEDICAL CENTERS
HARBORVIEW MEDICAL CENTER
UNIVERSITY OF WASHINGTON MEDICAL CENTER
SEATTLE, WASHINGTON

PAIN MANAGEMENT FLOWSHEET

UH 0827   SEP 89

EPIDURAL

PF Morphine

Fentanyl

Continuous infusion

Initials

Signature

Signature

Signature

Signature

113

APS PATIENT CONTROLLED ANALGESIA

ROYAL ADELAIDE HOSPITAL	**UR 72.2**
ACUTE PAIN SERVICE	Unit Record No.:
PATIENT CONTROLLED	Surname:
ANALGESIA (PCA)	Given Names:
Standard Orders	Date of Birth: _____ Sex: ___

1. No systemic opioid or sedatives to be given except as ordered by the APS.
2. Naloxone 400 microgram at bedside.
3. Oxygen at .... l/min via nasal specs or .... l/min via mask while orders in effect.
4. One-way antireflux valve to be used in IV line at all times.
5. **Monitoring and documentation:**

   a) Record pain score (at rest and with movement/coughing), sedation score, and respiratory rate hourly for 8 hours and then 2 hourly. Continue monitoring sedation score and respiratory rate (omit pain score) if asleep.

   b) After 48 hours the APS *only* may increase the monitoring interval. (*Date/time* .... *increase monitoring interval to 4 hourly. Signature of APS anaesthetist* ....)

   c) If sedation score ≥ 2 revert to hourly sedation scores until sedation score < 2 for 2 hours.

   d) Record current total dose at each monitoring interval. When the syringe is changed, check the machine settings and reset total dose to zero. Check settings at each shift change.

6. For inadequate analgesia or other problems related to PCA, contact the rostered APS anaesthetist. After 1800 hours this will be the on-call anaesthetic registrar.

7. **PCA ORDER:**

   a) Drug .... Route if other than IV ....

b) PCA settings:

* Loading dose = 0 (loading dose to be given prior to commencing PCA)

* Bolus dose = ... mg   * Dose duration = "stat"

* Lockout duration = 5 minutes   * Concentration = ... mg/ml

* Background infusion = ... mg/hr (........................ ml/hr)

c) If pain not controlled bolus dose may be increased to .... mg.

d) **If sedation score = 2, reduce size of the bolus dose by half and cease any background infusion.**

e) Cease PCA if the patient becomes confused.

8. **TREATMENT OF SIDE EFFECTS:**

a) **Respiratory depression**

If sedation score = 3 (irrespective of respiratory rate) <u>OR</u> sedation score = 2 <u>and</u> respiratory rate ≤ 6/minute, give 100 microgram NALOXONE IV stat. Repeat 2 minutely PRN up to a total of 400 microgram. Cease PCA and call the APS.

b) **Nausea/vomiting**

Give METOCLOPRAMIDE 10mg IV 4 hourly PRN. If ineffective, **add DROPERIDOL 500 mcg IV 4 hourly PRN (250 mcg if > 55 years old)**

9. **SIGNATURE OF ANAESTHETIST** .... Date ....

    (Print name..)

10. **Cease above orders**

    Signature of anaesthetist .... Date .... Time ....

CHAPTER 6

EPIDURAL AND INTRATHECAL ANALGESIA

Epidural analgesia is one of the most effective techniques available for the management of acute pain. It is particularly useful for the treatment of pain associated with activity, such as coughing or walking. In combination with active postoperative and post-injury rehabilitation protocols, epidural analgesia may lead to a reduction in postoperative complications (particularly respiratory and cardiac) and improved patient outcome, especially in the high-risk patient. The technique is associated with a number of uncommon but significant complications, so potential risks must always be weighed against possible advantages for each patient.

This form of pain relief will be initiated and managed by an anesthesiologist. If it is to be used after spinal surgery, the surgeon may place an epidural catheter at the end of the operation. Nevertheless, all medical staff must have an understanding of this form of analgesia in order to be aware of possible complications and drug interactions.

The availability of adequate and specialized care must always be considered. However, epidural and intrathecal analgesia can be safely managed on general hospital wards if the following are available:
- appropriate patient selection criteria
- appropriate standard orders and nursing procedure protocols
- nursing education and accreditation programs specific to epidural and intrathecal analgesia
- regular review of the patient by an anesthesiologist
- availability of an anesthesiologist at all times, for consultation or management of complications or inadequate pain relief
- agreement to delegate all responsibility for pain relief to one group of specialist medical staff (anesthesiologists) with consultation of this group by other medical personnel as required

ANATOMY

The spinal cord and brain are covered by three membranes, the meninges. The outer membrane is called the dura mater. The middle layer, the arachnoid, lies just below the dura and both form the dural sac. The inner layer, the pia mater, adheres to the surface of the spinal cord and brain. The *epidural space* lies between the dura mater and the bone and ligaments of the spinal canal (**Figure 6.1**). It is only a potential space containing blood vessels, nerve roots, fat and connective tissue. Deep to the arachnoid membrane is the subarachnoid or *intrathecal space*, containing cerebrospinal fluid (CSF) and the spinal cord above the level of L1–2 and the cauda equina (the lumbar and sacral nerve roots) below L1–2. The dural sac ends at S2.

To obtain *epidural analgesia*, analgesic drugs are administered directly into the epidural space. An epidural catheter is usually placed to enable repeated doses or an infusion of the drug to be given. Drugs administered directly into the CSF and used for *intrathecal analgesia* are more commonly given as a single dose

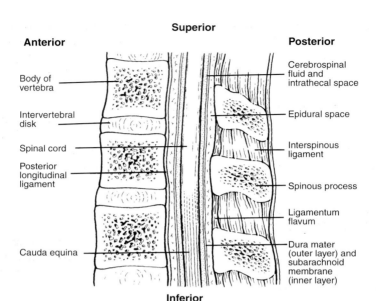

Superior

Anterior   **Posterior**

Body of vertebra

Intervertebral disk

Spinal cord

Posterior longitudinal ligament

Cauda equina

Cerebrospinal fluid and intrathecal space

Epidural space

Interspinous ligament

Spinous process

Ligamentum flavum

Dura mater (outer layer) and subarachnoid membrane (inner layer)

Inferior

Figure 6.1   Anatomy of the spinal cord

through a spinal needle at the time of spinal anesthesia. The doses of drugs required for intrathecal analgesia are much smaller than those required for epidural analgesia.

CONTRAINDICATIONS

The contraindications to epidural and intrathecal analgesia are summarized in **Box 6.1**.

UNTRAINED NURSING AND MEDICAL STAFF

Epidural and intrathecal analgesia should only be used in hospital wards where staff have received specific teaching about these methods of pain relief. Staff should have a good understanding of the techniques and monitoring requirements, and be able to recognize and treat (according to written orders) inadequate analgesia and side effects. Many institutions require some form of accreditation before nurses are allowed to take responsibility for patients with epidural or intrathecal analgesia. In addition, these methods of pain relief should only be used when an anesthesiologist is available to review patients daily and whenever problems arise.

PATIENT REJECTION

For many reasons patients may not want epidural or intrathecal analgesia. For example, they may have heard of possible complications, either from friends or from the media. A full explanation needs to be given to each patient and the risks and possible benefits explained.

CONTRAINDICATIONS TO THE PLACEMENT OF AN EPIDURAL NEEDLE OR CATHETER

There are a number of reasons why placement of an epidural needle or catheter might be contraindicated, or at least relatively contraindicated (i.e. potential benefits of placement may outweigh the risk).

Infection

Epidural needles and catheters should not be placed at the site of local infection. Generalized sepsis may increase the risk of an

Possible contraindications or relative contraindications to epidural and intrathecal analgesia

Untrained staff
Patient rejection
Contraindications to catheter or needle placement
• local or generalized sepsis
• some central or spinal neurological diseases
• hypovolemia
• coagulation disorders
• concurrent treatment with anticoagulant medications
Presence of a dural puncture

Box 6.1

epidural space infection and placement of an epidural catheter in such patients remains controversial. If the patient is receiving appropriate antibiotic cover and if the risk-benefit ratio has been considered, it may be appropriate in selected patients. The risk of performing epidural blockade in patients with human immunodeficiency virus (HIV) infection or acquired immune deficiency syndrome (AIDS) is unknown, as is the risk of blood patch for the treatment of postdural puncture headache in these patients.

Central nervous system disease

The decision to proceed with epidural analgesia in patients with diseases such as multiple sclerosis should be made on a case-by-case basis after an assessment of risks and benefits. One of the potential issues is that any exacerbation of the disease is likely to be blamed on the analgesic technique, whereas disease progression may have been coincidental.

Hypovolemia

The normal response to hypovolemia is peripheral vaso-constriction. If epidural local anesthetic drugs are given, the resultant vasodilatation may contribute to hypotension. Concurrent intravenous fluids and slow titration of the local anesthetic solution are recommended. The more dilute local anesthetic solutions may be less likely to contribute to postoperative hypotension.

Anticoagulants and coagulation disorders

In general, insertion of epidural or intrathecal needles and catheters should be avoided in patients with coagulation disorders or in those who are fully anticoagulated However, anticoagulant drugs may be given to patients with an epidural catheter already in place, as they are commonly prescribed for postoperative or post-trauma thromboprophylaxis. The risk of hematoma must be considered along with the potential benefits of epidural analgesia for each patient. Whenever possible, thromboprophylaxis can be instituted after the epidural catheter has been inserted and fixed in place.

Oral anticoagulants

There is little information about the risks of epidural hematoma in association with the use of warfarin. In patients on chronic warfarin therapy, hemostasis may require 4–6 days to normalize once the drug is stopped. Coagulation status should be checked before insertion of an epidural needle or catheter.

Some patients are prescribed low-dose warfarin for postoperative thromboprophylaxis (e.g. after major orthopedic surgery). The best time for removal of an epidural catheter in these patients is not known. In some centers, catheters are removed within 24–36 hours of the first postoperative dose; in others, the catheters are left in for longer periods. If this is done, monitoring of coagulation status is suggested. Up to 20% of patients may show some prolongation of prothrombin time after a single dose of warfarin.

Standard unfractionated heparin (intravenous)

Epidural catheterization appears to be relatively safe in patients who are heparinized either during or after surgery. However, consideration must be given to the timing of both needle and catheter placement *before* heparin is given and catheter removal *after* heparin is commenced. It has been suggested that epidural needles and catheters be placed at least 1–2 hours before heparin is given. In patients likely to receive large doses of heparin (e.g. during cardiac surgery) epidural catheters are sometimes sited the day before surgery. If a postoperative heparin infusion is required, the catheter should be removed after the infusion has been suspended for a few hours (after discussion with the treating physician). It may take 4–6 hours for activated partial thromboplastin times to decrease to suitable levels.

Standard unfractionated heparin (subcutaneous)

Low-dose standard heparin is commonly administered for thromboprophylaxis and is generally considered safe to use in patients with concurrent epidural analgesia. However, appropriate precautions should be taken regarding the timing of epidural catheter insertion and removal. The peak effect of a dose of standard heparin is likely to be seen at about 1 hour; duration of effect may be 4–6 hours or more. Despite the low doses (commonly 5000 U twice daily) a small number of patients will develop therapeutic plasma levels.

Low molecular weight heparin

In December 1997, the US Food and Drug Administration issued a public health advisory report regarding the risk of epidural hematoma in association with epidural and spinal anesthesia in patients receiving low molecular weight heparin (LMWH) as postoperative thromboprophylaxis.

Although LMWHs are used worldwide, the risk of epidural hematoma appeared to be much higher in the USA than in Europe. Reports from the USA concerned the LMWH enoxaparin, where the recommended dose after major joint replacement surgery was 30 mg twice a day. In Europe and Australasia, the recommended dose is 40 mg just once a day (20 mg only may be used for some nonorthopedic and lower risk patients). The higher risk in the USA may be a result of higher doses and a twice-daily dosing schedule, because a trough in anticoagulant activity between doses (which may allow for safer catheter removal) is less likely to occur.

The time to peak effect of a dose of LMWH is about 3–5 hours; normal hemostasis may not return until more than 12 hours after that dose. Therefore, the timing of epidural catheter insertion and removal must be considered carefully. These agents are excreted by the kidney and accumulation can occur in patients with renal impairment.

The concern about the risk of epidural hematoma in association with LMWH has led to the promulgation of a number of different guidelines. These are designed to suggest appropriate intervals between insertion and removal of epidural catheters relative to the time of LMWH administration. In the USA it has been recommended that LMWH should not be given earlier than 24 hours after surgery and that where possible, the catheter should be removed prior to initiation of therapy. In other countries with once-daily dose regimens, guidelines have often been less exacting, e.g. instituting the first dose of LMWH no sooner than 2 hours after catheter insertion and removing the catheter 1–2 hours before the next dose. Removal in the morning may allow easier monitoring of neurological function.

Despite the above suggestions, good evidence for exact intervals that will minimize risk is still lacking and most guidelines present a consensus view only. It is therefore likely that current guidelines will need revision as information and clinical practices evolve.

Monitoring of all patients receiving epidural analgesia (especially those where the possibility of abnormal coagulation exists) should include immediate reporting of new pain in the back or legs as well as any changes in neurological status.

Nonsteroidal anti-inflammatory drugs

The isolated use of nonsteroidal anti-inflammatory drugs (NSAIDs) including aspirin has not been identified as a risk factor for epidural hematoma. There is no generally accepted test that can reliably assess platelet function. However, concurrent use with other medications that affect coagulation status may increase the risk.

Thrombolytic therapy

In general, epidural analgesia should be avoided in patients receiving thrombolytic therapy (e.g. streptokinase) because of the increased risk of bleeding.

PRESENCE OF A DURAL PUNCTURE

If the dura has been punctured, either inadvertently during insertion of an epidural needle or catheter, or during spinal surgery, part of any drug injected into the epidural space may gain direct access to the CSF. The patient must be observed closely if a decision is made to proceed with epidural analgesia.

DRUGS USED FOR EPIDURAL ANALGESIA

Two classes of drugs are commonly used for epidural analgesia: opioids and local anesthetics. They can be given as repeated bolus doses or by continuous infusion and should be preservative-free. The doses and infusion rates suggested below are guidelines only and may vary according to patient age, medical condition, site of injection and other factors.

To improve both the quality and duration of analgesia, clonidine (an α_2-adrenergic agonist) or epinephrine (adrenaline) are sometimes added to local anesthetic or opioid solutions. The epidural use of other drugs for acute pain management (e.g. neostigmine and midazolam) still requires further investigation. Approval for the epidural administration of these drugs varies between countries.

OPIOIDS

Site of action

Epidural and intrathecal opioids produce analgesia by blocking opioid receptors in the dorsal horn of the spinal cord. When an opioid is injected into the epidural space, some is absorbed into the epidural blood vessels and enters the systemic circulation, some binds to epidural fat, and some crosses the dura and arachnoid membranes and enters the CSF.

The proportion of epidurally-administered opioid that is absorbed into the systemic circulation contributes to analgesia and to the development of opioid-related side effects. Plasma levels are highest after the administration of lipid-soluble opioids (e.g. fentanyl).

From the CSF a proportion of drug is taken up into the spinal cord. Bulk flow of CSF in a rostral direction means that any drug remaining in the CSF will be carried to spinal cord opioid receptors some distance from the site of injection. Rostral spread of drug has potential disadvantages as respiratory depression may occur if sufficient opioid remains in the CSF when it reaches the brain stem and the respiratory center. It can also contribute to the development of other side effects such as nausea, vomiting and pruritus.

Differences can be seen between opioids of low and high lipid solubility when onset of effect, duration of effect (**Box 6.2**) and side-effect profile are compared. Less lipid-soluble drugs (e.g. morphine) take longer to cross from the epidural space to CSF and have a slower onset of action. They are cleared more slowly from CSF, are more likely to spread rostrally, and have a longer duration of action.

The lipid-soluble drugs (e.g. fentanyl) are more rapid in onset, have a much shorter duration of action, are subject to greater vascular uptake from the epidural space, and have a more segmental spread and analgesic effect. The correct dermatomal positioning of the epidural catheter is therefore more important if lipid-soluble opioids are used.

Dosages

In general, the analgesic efficacy of opioids is greater when given epidurally compared with parenteral administration; that is, a smaller dose is needed in order to achieve the same or better

Epidural opioids: examples of bolus doses and infusion rates

Opioid	Bolus* (mg)	Onset (min)	Peak effect (min)	Dura- tion† (h)	Infu- sion* (mg/h)	Lipid solubility‡
Morphine	1–6	20–30	30–60	6–24	0.1–0.75	1
Hydromorphone	1–2	10–15	15–30	6–16	0.1–0.4	1.4
Diamorphine	2–6	5–10	10–15	6–12	0.2–1.0	280
Meperidine (pethidine)	20–50	5–10	15–30	1–6	10–30	39
Fentanyl	0.025–0.1	5–10	10–20	1–4	0.025–0.1	813
Sufentanil	0.01–0.05	5–10	10–15	1–6	0.01–0.05	1780

Box 6.2

*Effective doses will vary depending on patient age, medical condition and site of injection.

†Duration of analgesia varies widely; higher doses will have a longer duration of action.

‡Octanol/pH 7.4 buffer partition coefficient.

Values may vary according to diffrent references.

degree of pain relief. However, this varies according to the lipid solubility of the drug. Morphine, being the least lipid-soluble opioid used in epidural analgesia, shows the greatest difference in dose required by both routes to produce a similar analgesic effect (**Box 6.3**). With highly lipid-soluble drugs such as fentanyl, there is little or no difference.

Commonly used drugs, dosages, approximate rate of onset and duration of action, and infusion rates are listed in **Box 6.2**. Because of its more rapid onset, the use of a drug such as fentanyl can be useful in the event of breakthrough pain in a patient receiving epidural morphine.

Longer-acting opioids may be given by intermittent bolus dose or by infusion. Highly lipid-soluble opioids (e.g. fentanyl and sufentanil) are best administered by continuous infusion because of their short duration of action.

The total dose of opioid administered into the epidural space is the primary determinant of analgesic activity, but the volume in which the dose is administered may help to determine the spread of the dose. This is particularly so for more lipid-soluble opioids.

As with any opioid, the initial dose should be based on the age of the patient and subsequent doses titrated to effect. Morphine is commonly used when opioids alone are administered for epidural analgesia. Suggested initial doses via lumbar catheters for nonthoracic surgery or via thoracic catheters for thoracic surgery range from 4 mg in patients less than 45 years old to 1 mg in patients over 75 years old.

Approximate equianalgesic doses of morphine according to route of administration	
Oral	30 mg
Intramuscular	10 mg
Epidural	2–3 mg
Intrathecal	0.2–0.3 mg

Box 6.3

Side effects

Respiratory system

Respiratory depression is a possible complication of epidural opioids.

- *Early respiratory depression* usually occurs within 2 hours of an injection (or later with an infusion) and results from high blood levels of opioid following absorption from the epidural space into the systemic circulation.
- *Delayed respiratory depression* is most commonly seen 6–12 hours after the opioid was given and results from rostral migration of drug in the CSF to the brain stem and respiratory center. The onset is usually gradual with the patient becoming progressively more sedated. Delayed respiratory depression can persist for many hours. If naloxone is necessary it may have to be given by infusion.

Delayed respiratory depression is less likely with more lipid-soluble drugs (e.g. meperidine and fentanyl). Once in the CSF, these drugs are subject to rapid uptake into the spinal cord and blood vessels. The risk of significant concentrations of opioid reaching the respiratory center due to rostral spread is therefore much less than with morphine. However, the relatively high blood concentrations are more likely to cause early respiratory depression.

There is an increased risk of respiratory depression associated with:

- increasing patient age
- high doses of epidural (or intrathecal) opioid
- the opioid-naive patient
- concurrent use of sedatives or systemic opioids (including long-acting sedatives or large doses of parenteral opioid given before or during an operation)

As with other methods of opioid administration, a decrease in respiratory rate can be a late and unreliable sign of respiratory depression. Therefore, frequent assessments of patient sedation should be made. If a patient becomes excessively sedated, subsequent bolus doses should be reduced and infusions stopped or decreased. Naloxone may be required (see **Box 6.9**).

commonly used for anesthesia (e.g. 0.125–0.25% bupivacaine, 0.2% ropivacaine). The suggested infusion rates are similar to those prescribed for local anesthetic – opioid combinations (see **Box 6.5**).

Side effects

Local neurotoxicity or systemic toxicity (due to inadvertent overdose or intravascular injection) may follow epidural administration of local anesthetics (for details refer to Chapter 3). A 'total spinal', with unconsciousness and cardiovascular collapse, can occur if excessive doses are inadvertently given intrathecally.

Blockade of autonomic and motor fibers as well as sensory nerves may result in other side effects including the following.

Respiratory system

The diaphragm is the most important muscle of involuntary respiration. It is supplied by cervical nerves 3 to 5, which are unlikely to be blocked by the usual volumes and concentrations of local anesthetic drug used for epidural anesthesia and analgesia. Dense motor block of intercostal muscles can reduce a patient's ability to take a deep breath and cough. However, the degree of block that occurs with the low concentrations of local anesthetic normally used for postoperative analgesia is clinically insignificant.

Cardiovascular system

Sympathetic block can lead to hypotension. The greater the number of segments blocked and the higher the concentration and total dose of epidural local anesthetic administered, the greater the chance of hypotension.

In the low concentrations normally used in combination with opioids for pain relief on general wards, significant hypotension is unlikely unless the patient is also hypovolemic. However, even partial sympathetic blockade may prevent compensatory mechanisms from being fully effective. Postural or orthostatic hypotension is therefore possible.

If hypotension occurs it will normally respond to intravenous fluids but vasopressors (such as ephedrine) may be required.

These should be available in all wards where epidural local anesthetic agents or local anesthetic/opioid mixtures are used.

If the block extends above T4 (nipple line) and if enough local anesthetic solution has been given, the cardioaccelerator fibers to the heart may be blocked, leading to bradycardia. Bradycardia may respond to atropine. If bradycardia or hypotension is severe, epinephrine (adrenaline) may be more effective.

Sedation

Unless local anesthetic doses are large there is unlikely to be significant sedation.

Nausea and vomiting

Nausea and vomiting are much less common following epidural local anesthetics than epidural opioids.

Pruritus

Pruritus is not a side effect of epidural local anesthetic agents.

Motor/sensory block

Immobility is not desirable after injury or surgery, so low concentrations of local anesthetic drug are often used in an attempt to preferentially block smaller sensory fibers while avoiding a block of the larger motor fibers (*differential block*: see Chapter 3). Motor block and difficulty with walking are less likely to occur with thoracic epidural blockade compared with lumbar placement of the catheter.

By using an infusion of low concentrations of local anesthetic drug in combination with an opioid, effective analgesia can often be achieved with a minimum of motor block or block of other sensory nerves. If a patient complains of numbness or weakness, the infusion can be stopped for a short while and then restarted at a lower rate. If the problem persists the concentration of local anesthetic drug may be reduced or the technique changed to use of an epidural opioid only. Numbness and weakness may also be the first signs of catheter migration into CSF, epidural abscess or epidural hematoma (see later).

Patients receiving epidural infusions of a local anesthetic (or local anesthetic and opioid) can often sit out of bed or walk about. However, this should be done slowly and with assistance because of the risks of leg weakness, loss of position sense or postural hypotension.

Pressure areas have been reported following epidural analgesia, presumably due to a combination of immobility and decreased sensation. Care must also be taken in patients at risk of compartment syndrome, when epidural analgesia could mask early signs and symptoms of this complication. In some patients epidural analgesia may be best avoided; in others it is important to avoid motor or significant sensory blockade.

Urinary retention

As with epidural opioids urinary retention can occur but is not inevitable, and does not require routine prophylactic catheterization.

Gastrointestinal system

Bowel motility is unimpaired or even improved. This allows for quicker recovery of gastrointestinal function after abdominal surgery. This benefit is more likely to be seen in patients who have thoracic epidural catheters placed for analgesia, compared with those in whom lumbar catheters are inserted. Concerns about an increased risk of anastomotic breakdown due to increased intestinal motility appear to be unfounded, and epidural analgesia using local anesthetic drugs is generally considered to be safe for patients undergoing bowel resection with an anastomosis. Earlier return of motility is also seen when opioid is added to the local anesthetic solution, compared with epidural opioid alone.

COMBINATIONS OF LOCAL ANESTHETIC AND OPIOID AGENTS

The side effects of opioid and local anesthetic agents used in epidural analgesia are compared in **Box 6.4**.

In an attempt to minimize the adverse effects of each class of drug and provide better analgesia than that attained with either agent alone, a combination of an opioid and a low concentration of local anesthetic solution (colloquially called an 'epidural cocktail') is often given by continuous infusion. This combination is more effective than epidural opioids alone and the effect appears to be synergistic.

While the aim of the combination therapy is to obtain the full benefits of each class of drug before side effects from either class occur, optimal concentrations of each remain unknown. The following are examples of commonly used mixtures:

- 0.0625% bupivacaine and 2 µg/ml fentanyl (or 20 µg/ml morphine)
- 0.1% bupivacaine and 5 µg/ml fentanyl (or 40 µg/ml morphine)
- 0.125% bupivacaine and 5 µg/ml fentanyl (or 40 µg/ml morphine)

Infusions of 0.2% ropivacaine and 2–5 µg/ml fentanyl have also been shown to be effective. Other opioids that have been used in

Comparison of the possible side effects of epidural opioids and local anesthetic drugs

	Opioid	Local anesthetic
Respiratory	Delayed depression Early depression	Usually unimpaired
Cardiovascular	Usually no reduction in blood pressure	Overt or postural hypotension Reduced heart rate with high block
Sedation	Yes	Mild/absent
Nausea/vomiting	Yes	Less common
Pruritus	Yes	No
Motor	No effect	Block
Sensation	No effect	Block
Urinary retention	Yes	Yes
Gastrointestinal	Decreased motility	Increased motility

Box 6.4
Adapted from Cousins and Mather (1984).

combination with bupivacaine include meperidine (pethidine), diamorphine and sufentanil. It is the total dose of drugs given that is important; the higher the concentration the lower the volume infused. The siting of the epidural catheter, in the middle of the dermatomal segments to be covered, is important when a combination of drugs is used.

Dose regimens

Infusion rates will vary according to the concentration of drugs in the solutions, the site of injury or surgery relative to the site of epidural catheter placement, and the age of the patient. In institutions where nursing staff are allowed to administer 'top-up' doses as well as alter infusion rates, orders should include bolus doses of the solution for breakthrough pain. Suggested bolus doses and infusion rates for some of the bupivacaine/fentanyl combinations that may be used are listed in **Box 6.5**.

STANDARD ORDERS AND NURSING PROCEDURE PROTOCOLS

Standard orders and nursing procedure protocols are recommended to maximize the safety and effectiveness of epidural analgesia. To reduce the risk of drugs or fluids intended for intravenous (IV) administration being inadvertently given via an epidural catheter, all catheters should carry a clearly visible label.

STANDARD ORDERS

To standardize orders throughout the institution, preprinted forms are recommended. The forms need to be completed, signed and dated by the treating anesthesiologist. Examples of preprinted epidural standard orders are provided at the end of this chapter.

It should be noted that while standard orders are used for the initial prescription of epidural analgesia, these orders may not be effective for all patients. Daily evaluation (or more often if required) of the patient by an anesthesiologist will allow appropriate alterations to be made to the prescription or analgesic technique. Daily assessment should usually include:

	Younger patients **(up to 40 years)**	**to**	**Older patients** **(over 70 years)**
Infusion rate (ml/h)	8–15	to	4–8
PRN bolus doses (ml)	4–8	to	2–4

Suggestions for initial infusion rates and bolus doses using 0.0625% to 0.1% bupivacaine and 2–5 µg/ml fentanyl

Box 6.5
- these doses may also vary according to other factors such as site of catheter placement and height of patient
- thoracic epidural infusions may require slightly smaller volumes than lumbar epidural infusions
- lower infusion rates are needed if higher concentrations of drug are used

- effectiveness of analgesia at rest and with activity
- effectiveness of the treatment of any side effects
- evaluation of any clinical features than might suggest a catheter-related complication
- an overall assessment of the patient, including the possibility of non-analgesia-related complications, and any concurrent medication orders

Standard orders need to cover a number of different areas, as follows:

Nondrug treatment orders
Nondrug treatment orders may include a statement to eliminate the concurrent ordering of CNS depressants or other opioids by others, orders for oxygen, maintenance of IV access, and instructions as to whom to contact if problems occur.

Monitoring and documentation requirements
The following should be monitored at regular intervals:

- pain score, sedation score and respiratory rate
- blood pressure and heart rate (which should be recorded for at least the first 24 hours if local anesthetic drugs are used)
- sensory block – block height may be measured by testing the level at which the patient reports a change in sensation from cold to warmth when ice or alcohol is applied to the skin. However, the differences may not be very marked when low concentrations of local anesthetic drug are infused and routine monitoring of sensory block height may not be required or possible in this circumstance. Any sensory deficit should, however, be noted
- motor block – the ability of a patient to raise a straight leg will provide evidence that lower extremity motor block is not excessive

All observations should be documented (see the examples of flowsheets at the end of Chapter 5) at regular intervals (hourly for up to 24 hours and then 2- to 4-hourly is suggested), along with total amount of drug delivered, dose of any drug administered for the treatment of side effects and any changes that have been made to the infusion rates.

Drug orders
Orders for drug doses, drug concentrations, dose intervals or infusion rates, and instructions for the treatment of inadequate analgesia are required.

Orders for the treatment of side effects
The inclusion of standard orders for the recognition and management of side effects will minimize delays in treatment.

NURSING PROCEDURE PROTOCOLS
The format of nursing procedure protocols for epidural analgesia will vary with each institution, but there are elements that need to be included in each, regardless of format. These are listed in **Box 6.6**.

Elements to be included in nursing procedure protocols for epidural analgesia

- a statement of institution policy towards accreditation for nursing staff responsible for a patient with epidural or intrathecal analgesia
- a statement indicating who has responsibility for writing epidural or intrathecal orders
- mechanisms for the checking and discarding of opioids
- guidelines for the suitability, or otherwise, of patients for epidural or intrathecal analgesia
- guidelines for preoperative patient education (the technique should also be explained to the patient in detail by the anesthesiologist)
- monitoring and documentation requirements
- instructions for administration of bolus doses (including the need to aspirate the catheter using a small syringe to check for presence of CSF or blood)
- instructions for checking the amount of drug delivered (from the infusion pump display) against the amount remaining in the syringe
- detailed instruction on the setting up and programming of infusion pumps and the management of equipment faults and alarms
- instructions for checking the catheter insertion site, redressing of the site if needed and for the labeling of the epidural catheters
- instructions for checking and documenting completeness of epidural catheter tip once removed (catheters may be removed by anesthesiologists in some institutions)
- instructions for mobilization of the patient (mobilization should be encouraged)
- instructions about whom to call if assistance or advice is required

Box 6.6

SUBSEQUENT ANALGESIC REGIMENS

Unlike PCA, epidural doses cannot be used as a guide for the prescription of subsequent analgesic regimens. If opioids are prescribed (parenteral or oral) appropriate age-based doses are suggested (see Chapter 4).

There should be some overlap of pain therapies so that the subsequent regimen has time to have an effect before the first is withdrawn. If there is to be a change in clinical responsibility for the pain management of the patient, then this change needs to be clearly understood by all staff.

COMPLICATIONS OF EPIDURAL ANALGESIA

Complications of epidural analgesia may be related to the epidural needle or catheter, the equipment, or side effects of the drugs (**Box 6.7**). Management of complications related to the insertion of a needle or catheter is summarized in **Box 6.8**.

POSTDURAL PUNCTURE HEADACHE

Whenever the dura is punctured, intentionally or unintentionally, leakage of CSF can occur. This can lead to a decrease in CSF pressure and tension on meningeal vessels and nerves, which can result in headache. The risk of dural puncture is estimated to be about 0.16–1.3%, with the subsequent risk of headache ranging from 16% to 86%. It is less with smaller needles, certain types of needles and in older patients.

The signs and symptoms are fairly typical and usually occur 1–2 days after the puncture. The headache is usually bifrontal and/or occipital, worse if the patient sits or strains, and may be

Possible complications of epidural analgesia

Related to the insertion of an epidural needle or catheter:
- postdural puncture headache
- nerve or spinal cord injury
- epidural hematoma
- epidural space infection/meningitis
- catheter migration

Related to the equipment:
- catheter/filter
- infusion pumps

Related to the use of opioid and/or local anesthetic drugs

Inadequate analgesia

Box 6.7

Management of complications related to insertion of epidural needles or catheters*

Dural puncture headache
- bed rest
- analgesia (simple or opioid)
- hydrate (oral or IV)
- blood patch

Nerve or spinal cord injury
- immediate neurological assessment

Epidural space infection or hematoma
- immediate neurosurgical assessment
- MRI scan (contrast CT if no MRI)
- urgent surgical decompression if neurological changes develop due to nerve or spinal cord compression
- antibiotics (where appropriate)

Epidural catheter migration
- treat as for complications of excessive opioid and/or local anesthetic doses

Box 6.8
   *These strategies are suggestions only and may not be needed in, or suitable for, the treatment of all patients.

associated with nausea and vomiting, photophobia, depression and tinnitus. Severe cases may be associated with diplopia or other cranial nerve palsies, resulting from traction on these nerves. Very rarely, intracranial bleeding has resulted.

Initial treatment consists of bed rest, hydration and analgesia (simple or opioid). In some centers caffeine has been used with success. If these measures are not effective a 'blood patch' can be performed. This means that another epidural needle is inserted and, in a sterile manner, 10 ml of the patient's blood is injected into the epidural space. This effectively seals the hole through which the CSF is leaking. Relief from the headache is almost immediate in 95% of cases. Blood patches may occasionally cause minor backache or headache.

should be presumed to indicate epidural hematoma (or abscess – see below) until proved otherwise. Temporary cessation of the infusion may be appropriate until it can be shown that these signs will resolve.

It is also important for the patient to be aware of the need to report any motor or sensory changes as well as alterations in bladder or bowel function.

EPIDURAL SPACE INFECTION

Infections of the epidural space are also uncommon complications of epidural analgesia. Infection may result from direct needle or catheter inoculation, infusion of contaminated fluid, hematogenous spread during episodes of bacteremia, or by tracking of a superficial infection at the site of insertion along the catheter to the epidural space. The last is probably the most common source as the majority of infections are caused by various *Stapylococcus* organisms. As with epidural hematomas, infections can occur spontaneously (estimated to account for up to 2 in 10 000 hospital admissions). If an abscess develops, nerve root or spinal cord compression may result. Meningitis has also been reported.

Diagnosis

The signs and symptoms of an epidural abscess may be similar to those of an epidural hematoma, except that onset is often later and slower. The most frequent presenting symptoms are increasing and persistent back pain, back tenderness and signs of infection. If neurological signs develop, they may be delayed until some days later, although this is not always the case. Presentation of an epidural abscess may be delayed until days or weeks after the patient has been discharged from hospital.

The MRI scan is superior to other methods of imaging and should be the diagnostic test of choice if available (with or without contrast enhancement). Computed tomographic scans have given false or inconclusive findings, although reliability may be improved if contrast enhancement is used.

Patients with meningitis may present with fever, severe headache, photophobia, neck stiffness and altered levels of consciousness. A lumbar puncture should be performed to confirm the diagnosis (but not if an abscess is suspected, as contamination of the intrathecal space may result).

Treatment

An urgent neurosurgical consultation should be requested. In the absence of neurological complications, epidural space infections have been successfully treated with antibiotics. However, the development of any neurological changes indicates the need for an urgent neurosurgical consultation, as surgical decompression within 8–12 hours of onset of neurological signs and symptoms will allow the best chance of full recovery.

Prevention

As with an epidural hematoma, it may not be possible to prevent the development of an epidural space infection, but every attempt should be made to minimize the risk. For example, the catheter should always be inserted using an aseptic technique and epidural infusion solutions should be prepared under sterile conditions. Possible patient-related risk factors include sepsis, diabetes, depressed immune status, steroid therapy and alcohol abuse. If epidural analgesia is to be used in these patients, an assessment of risk versus benefit should, as always, be made. Duration of catheterization is not a good predictor of risk and epidural infections have been reported as soon as one day after insertion of an epidural catheter.

It is possible to maximize the chance of early detection of an abscess if epidural analgesia is used in a way that does not mask the onset of neurological changes, and if staff maintain a high index of suspicion. Should infection occur, early recognition and treatment will reduce the chance of more serious and permanent sequelae. The approach outlined above for epidural hematomas should be followed. In addition, the epidural catheter insertion site should be inspected daily and note taken of the patient's temperature. The catheter should usually be removed if inflammation or tenderness at the insertion site are present. Significant local infection should be treated with the appropriate antibiotics and surgical drainage may be required. If the patient develops a fever greater than would be expected in the immediate postoperative period, consideration may be given to removal of the catheter, unless the perceived benefit of continuing outweighs possible risks.

There appears to be little benefit from routine culture of epidural catheter tips after removal, as the positive culture may be as high as 30%. This presumably results from contamination of the tip upon removal and the results are therefore not reliable predictors of epidural space infection.

Patient education and involvement are again important. Patients must be instructed to report to the hospital or their anesthesiologist immediately if any problems are noted after discharge. An information sheet to be taken home may serve as a reminder (some examples are given at the end of Chapter 12).

CATHETER MIGRATION

Rarely a catheter placed in the epidural space will migrate into the intrathecal space or an epidural blood vessel. If migration is not recognized, large doses of drugs (opioids and/or local anesthetics) intended for epidural administration will be delivered into the CSF or systemic circulation. Complications due to catheter migration will be more obvious and of greater magnitude if bolus doses of epidural opioid and/or local anesthetic drug are given.

PROBLEMS RELATED TO EQUIPMENT

Epidural catheter or filter

Disconnection of the catheter from the epidural filter can result in contamination of the end of the catheter and migration of bacteria in the epidural infusion solution. If this disconnection is witnessed and it is important for epidural analgesia to continue, it may be reasonable to reconnect the catheter after the outside of the catheter has been thoroughly cleaned with an antiseptic solution and 10–20 cm trimmed from its end with sterile scissors. This should not be done without consulting the anesthesiologist responsible for the epidural analgesia.

Kinking of the catheter can occur, making infusion or administration of a bolus dose difficult or impossible. The length of the catheter should be checked for obvious kinks; if none is visible it may be worth pulling the catheter back by 1–2 cm (time of any heparin administration allowing). Slight flexion of the patient's back may also overcome the problem.

Leaking filters should be replaced as there is a risk of contamination of the epidural solution. If the catheter appears to be leaking at the insertion site it may be that the tip of the catheter is no longer in the epidural space but lying in subcutaneous tissue. In this case, analgesia is likely to be inadequate. If analgesia appears to be adequate, treatment may be continued.

The catheter should be inspected on removal to ensure that the tip is complete. If it is not, the patient should be told and details entered in the patient's record. The catheter material is inert and surgical removal of the tip is usually unnecessary.

Infusion pumps

Operator error can lead to misprogramming of infusion pumps, infusion pumps may malfunction, or patients may attempt to interfere with the running of the pumps. Unlike PCA machines, drugs contained in most infusion or syringe pumps are easily accessible to all.

Fatal or near-fatal doses of epidural analgesic drugs have been given when infusion pumps delivering the epidural solution have been mistakenly programmed to the rate prescribed for the infusion of intravenous fluids. A wide variety of drugs intended for intravenous administration has also been injected or infused into the epidural space. Consideration should be given to the clear labeling of all epidural catheters and infusion devices used for epidural analgesia.

Excessive doses of epidural infusion solutions have also been administered when the contents of a syringe or infusion bag have accidentally been allowed to empty by gravity. Therefore, infusion devices should be placed at an appropriate level relative to the patient.

SIDE EFFECTS RELATED TO THE DRUGS

Possible side effects of epidural and intrathecal opioids and local anesthetic agents were outlined earlier in this chapter (see **Box**

Management of side effects of epidural analgesia*

Nausea/vomiting
- administer antiemetics (change if ineffective)
- decrease the size of the bolus dose or the rate of the epidural infusion
- consider other possible causes
- change to another opioid
- lie patient flat and minimize movement until treatment has had time to work

Pruritus
- change to another opioid
- administer small doses of IV naloxone or an opioid agonist-antagonist (e.g. nalbuphine)
- ? administer an antihistamine (watch for sedation)

Sedation and respiratory depression
- sedation score 2, respiratory rate > 8/min: reduce the size of bolus doses and/or the rate of infusion
- sedation score 2, respiratory rate < 8/min: reduce the bolus dose and/or infusion rate, consider naloxone
- sedation score 3 (regardless of respiratory rate): administer naloxone and stop the infusion
- a decrease in opioid concentration may be required

Urinary retention
- try small doses of IV naloxone (if opioid only being used)
- catheterize – 'in-out' or indwelling

Hypotension
- look for causes of hypovolemia
- administer IV fluids +/– vasopressors
- cease/reduce (often only temporarily) infusion

Numbness/weakness (local anesthetic +/– opioid)
- check for catheter migration (into CSF)
- cease infusion for a short while, restart at a lower rate once there is evidence of resolution of sensory and motor deficit
- consider reducing local anesthetic concentration if above fails

Box 6.9
*These strategies are suggestions only and may not be needed in, or suitable for, the treatment of all patients.

6.4). Side effects will be exaggerated if doses intended for epidural administration are inadvertently given directly into the CSF. Suggestions for the management of these complications are listed in **Box 6.9**.

Care must be taken to ensure a bolus dose of the epidural analgesic solution is not inadvertently administered during the changing of any syringes. Drug-related problems may also occur if there are errors in prescription – either by mistake or due to inadequate knowledge.

INADEQUATE ANALGESIA

In general, it is best to establish epidural anesthesia using stronger concentrations of local anesthetic agent before the lower-concentration local anesthetic/opioid solutions used for analgesia are commenced. The analgesic infusion can be started before the initial block has regressed completely. Continued resolution of motor and sensory blockade will usually proceed despite the infusion of a lower-concentration solution. Reduction in intensity of motor and sensory block, as well as satisfactory analgesia, should be evident before the patient is transferred to a general ward.

If a patient complains of inadequate pain relief, assessment must first consider causes other than the site of operation or injury. Examples include pain resulting from a postoperative complication, pain at sites distant to the incision and related to the surgery but not covered by epidural analgesia (e.g. shoulder tip pain following laparoscopic or thoracic surgery), or a patient with an epidural placed for pain from fractured ribs but with painful injuries at other sites also. In some situations additional analgesia may be required. If other opioids are needed in addition to epidural analgesia (e.g. by PCA) it may be appropriate to use local anesthetic drugs only in the epidural infusion, so that opioids are given by one route only (in order to minimize the risk of respiratory depression).

If pain appears to be related to the surgery, the procedures outlined in **Box 6.10** can be tried.

Suggestions for the management of inadequate epidural analgesia*

- give a bolus dose of opioid or opioid/local anesthetic solution and increase the rate of an infusion
- check position of catheter using a 'test dose' of 3–8 ml of local anesthetic solution (e.g. 1% lidocaine or 0.25% bupivacaine) and test for level of sensory block ('test dose' to be administered by an anesthesiologist only)
- evidence of a bilateral block indicates need for increased dose (increased infusion rate or concentration of local anesthetic)
- if block is unilateral the catheter tip may have exited the epidural space through an intervertebral foramen. Withdraw catheter or try a larger bolus dose (note time of any heparin administration)
- If 'test dose' shows no block the catheter is displaced – order alternative analgesia or reinsert catheter (note time of last dose of heparin)

Box 6.10

*These strategies are suggestions only and may not be needed in, or suitable for, the treatment of all patients.

PATIENT-CONTROLLED EPIDURAL ANALGESIA

Although epidural analgesia has been shown to provide superior pain relief, patient satisfaction is often higher with intravenous patient-controlled analgesia (IV-PCA). Patient-controlled epidural analgesia (PCEA) combines the benefits of more effective analgesia with the advantages of patient control. Experience with PCEA for the management of acute pain is still limited, but both opioids and combinations of opioid and local anesthetic drugs have been used.

As with IV-PCA, a loading dose should be given before PCEA is commenced. Unlike IV-PCA, a continuous (background) infusion is more commonly ordered. The parameters that have been used by some groups are listed in **Box 6.11**.

Patient-controlled epidural analgesia: examples of parameters used

Drug	Bolus dose (mg)	Lock-out interval (min)	Background infusion (mg/h)
Morphine	0.2	10	+/– 0.4
Meperidine (pethidine)	10–30	5–20	+/– 30
Fentanyl	0.015–0.05	5–15	+/– 0.05–0.1
Sufentanil	0.004	6	+/– 0.008
Hydromorphone	0.15–0.3	15–30	
Bupivacaine 0.05–0.125% + 1–5 µg/ml fentanyl	2–5 ml	10–20	+/– 3–6 ml/h

Box 6.11

INTRATHECAL ANALGESIA

The contraindications, complications and the management of complications of intrathecal analgesia are similar to epidural analgesia. Standard orders and nursing procedure protocols are also recommended.

DRUGS USED FOR INTRATHECAL ANALGESIA

Opioids alone (i.e. not a combination of local anesthetic and opioid) are commonly used for intrathecal analgesia in acute pain management. The opioid is delivered directly into the CSF, avoiding absorption by epidural fat and blood vessels. Rostral migration in the CSF will occur, particularly with morphine.

DOSES

The doses of opioids administered intrathecally are much smaller than doses required for epidural analgesia. As with epidural opioid analgesia, the more lipid-soluble the drug the more rapid the onset and the shorter the duration of action.

The drugs listed in **Box 6.12** have all been used for intrathecal analgesia. Because meperidine (pethidine) has local anesthetic as well as opioid properties, it has been used as the sole spinal anesthetic agent (in larger doses of 30–50 mg) for a variety of lower limb operations.

Although most intrathecal opioids are given as a 'once only' dose at the time of spinal anesthesia, a catheter may occasionally be left in place. All spinal catheters must be clearly labeled to distinguish them from epidural catheters.

POSSIBLE SIDE EFFECTS

Side effects are similar to those that occur with epidural opioids. Although some believe that the incidence is higher with intrathecal opioids, this is, to a large extent, dose-dependent.

If respiratory depression occurs following administration of intrathecal morphine, the time of peak risk is about 8–10 hours after injection. Respiratory depression appears to peak 5–20 minutes following intrathecal administration of highly lipophilic drugs. Increasing patient age, high doses of intrathecal opioid, an opioid-naive patient and concurrent use of sedatives or systemic opioids are associated with an increased risk of respiratory depression.

Intrathecal opioids: examples of doses used

Opioid	Dose (mg)	Onset (min)	Duration (h)
Morphine	0.1–0.5	15–30	8–24
Meperidine (pethidine)	10–25	5–10	6–12
Fentanyl	0.006–0.05	<10	1–4
Sufentanil	0.005–0.02	<10	2–6
Diamorphine	0.5–1	<10	10–20

Box 6.12

MANAGEMENT OF INADEQUATE ANALGESIA

Usually intrathecal opioids are administered as a single dose so that if analgesia is inadequate, supplementation with oral or parenteral opioids will be required. As this may increase the risk of respiratory depression, smaller than average doses (e.g. half the normal size bolus doses for PCA) should be administered initially and increased only if they prove to be inadequate.

REFERENCES AND FURTHER READING

Ballantyne J.C., Carr D.B., deFerranti S. et al. (1998) The comparative effects of postoperative analgesic therapies on pulmonary outcome: cumulative meta-analyses of randomized, controlled trials. *Anesthesia and Analgesia* **86**, 598–612.

Breivik H. (1998) Neurological complications in association with spinal and epidural analgesia – again. *Acta Anaesthesiologica Scandinavica* **42**, 609–613.

Breivik H. (1999) Infectious complications of epidural anaesthesia and analgesia. *Current Opinion in Anaesthesiology* **12**, 573–577.

Chaney M. (1995) Side effects of intrathecal and epidural opioids. *Canadian Journal of Anaesthesia* **42**, 891–903.

Cousins M.J. and Mather L.E. (1984) Intrathecal and epidural administration of opioids. *Anesthesiology* **61**, 276–310.

De Leon-Casasola O.A. and Lema M.J. (1996). Postoperative epidural opioid analgesia: what are the choices? *Anesthesia and Analgesia* **83**, 867–875.

Duffy P.J. and Crosby E.T. (1999) The epidural blood patch: resolving the controversies. *Canadian Journal of Anaesthesia* **46**, 878–886.

Hamber E.A. and Viscomi C.M. (1999) Intrathecal lipophilic opioids as adjuncts to surgical spinal anesthesia. *Regional Anesthesia and Pain Medicine* **24**, 255–263.

Horlocker T.T. and Wedel D.J. (2000) Neurological complications of spinal and epidural anesthesia. *Regional Anesthesia and Pain Medicine* **25**, 83–98.

Kindler C.H., Seeberger M.D. and Staender S.E. (1998) Epidural abscess complicating epidural anesthesia and analgesia: an analysis of the literature. *Acta Anaesthesiologica Scandinavica* **42**, 614–620.

Liu S., Carpenter R.L. and Neal J.M. (1995) Epidural anesthesia and analgesia: their role in postoperative outcome. *Anesthesiology* **82**, 1474–1506.

Meifssner A., Rolf N. and Van Aken H. (1997) Thoracic epidural anesthesia and the patient with heart disease: risks and controversies. *Anesthesia and Analgesia* **85**, 517–528.

National Health and Medical Research Council (1999) *Acute Pain Management: The Scientific Evidence.* Canberra (available at http://www.nhmrc.health.gov.au/publicat/pdf/cp57.pdf).

Neuraxial anesthesia and anticoagulation (1998) *Regional Anesthesia and Pain Medicine* **23**, suppl. 2 (all articles in this issue of the journal relate to the use of anticoagulants in neuraxial blockade).

Niemi G. and Breivik H. (1999) Adrenaline markedly improves thoracic epidural analgesia produced by low-dose infusion of bupivacaine, fentanyl and adrenaline after major surgery. *Acta Anaesthesiologica Scandinavica* **42**, 897–909.

Ready L.B., Ashburn M., Caplan R.A. et al. (1994) Practice guidelines for acute pain management in the perioperative setting – a report of the American Society of Anesthesiologists Task Force on Pain Management, Acute Pain Section. *Anesthesiology* **82**, 1071–1081

Ready L.B., Chadwick H.S. and Ross B. (1987) Age predicts effective epidural morphine dose after abdominal hysterectomy. *Anesthesia and Analgesia* **66**, 1215–1218.

Simpson R.S., Macintyre P.E., Shaw D. et al. (2000) Epidural catheter tip cultures: results of a 4-year audit and implications for clinical practice. *Regional Anesthesia and Pain Medicine* **25**, 360–367.

Steinbrook R. (1998) Epidural anesthesia and gastrointestinal motility. *Anesthesia and Analgesia* **86**, 831–844.

US Food and Drug Administration (1997) *FDA Public Health Advisory Committee report.* December 15 (available at http://www.fda.gov).

Vandermeulen E. (1999) Is anticoagulation and central neural blockade a safe combination? *Current Opinion in Anaesthesiology* **12**, 539–543.

APPENDIX TO CHAPTER 6

Examples of standard orders for epidural analgesia, reproduced with permission of the Acute Pain Services at the Royal Adelaide Hospital, Adelaide, Australia and the University of Washington Medical Center, Seattle, Washington, USA.

6A Royal Adelaide Hospital Acute Pain Service epidural/intrathecal/regional analgesia standard orders

6B University of Washington Medical Center Acute Pain Service epidural analgesia physician orders

KEEP AT BEDSIDE:
NALOXONE 0.4 mg

KEEP AT BEDSIDE:
NALOXONE 0.4 mg
EPHEDRINE 25 mg/5 ml (i.e. 5 mg/ml)

1. Maintain IV access (drip or peripheral lock with flushes) until epidural analgesia discontinued.
2. **No narcotics or other CNS depressants** to be given except as ordered by Acute Pain Service.
3. **Epidural Analgesia not to be discontinued** except by the Acute Pain Service.
4. **PRN Treatments:**

   A. NALOXONE 0.4 mg **IV stat** for sedation scale = 3 **plus** RR < 8 per minute. Call Acute Pain Service.
   B. METOCLOPRAMIDE 10 mg IV q 4 h prn for nausea/vomiting. **In addition, if age < 60 years**, TRANSDERMAL SCOPOLAMINE PATCH to either mastoid area. Change q 72 h prn.
   C. DIPHENHYDRAMINE 25 mg, IV or PO q 6 h prn for severe itching.
   D. For urinary retention, "in and out" bladder catheter prn.
   E. If age < 60 years, TRIAZOLAM 0.125 mg PO qhs prn. MR x 1.

Dr. _____ on the Acute Pain Service was notified about this patient at _____ hours.

DATE	TIME	PHYSICIAN SIGNATURE

UNIVERSITY OF WASHINGTON MEDICAL CENTERS
HARBORVIEW MEDICAL CENTER
UNIVERSITY OF WASHINGTON MEDICAL CENTER
SEATTLE, WASHINGTON

ACUTE PAIN SERVICE EPIDURAL ANALGESIA PHYSICIAN ORDERS

UH 0949 REV NOV 92

WHITE - MEDICAL RECORD
CANARY - PHARMACY
PINK - NURSING

PT.NO.

NAME

D.O.B.

CHAPTER 7

OTHER DRUGS USED IN ACUTE PAIN MANAGEMENT

◆

Nonsteroidal anti-inflammatory drugs

NMDA receptor antagonist drugs

Alpha-2-adrenergic agonist drugs

Nitrous oxide

Drugs other than opioids and local anesthetic agents may be used in the treatment of acute pain, either as the sole agent or as adjuvant medication. Some of these drugs (e.g. tricyclic antidepressants, anticonvulsants) are used primarily in the management of neuropathic pain and are discussed in Chapter 10.

NONSTEROIDAL ANTI-INFLAMMATORY DRUGS

The analgesic and anti-inflammatory properties of the bark of willow and other plants have been known for centuries. The active ingredient in willow bark is *salicin*, which can be converted to salicylic acid. Most compounds obtained from natural sources are expensive and have therefore been replaced by synthetic salicylates and other nonsteroidal anti-inflammatory drugs (NSAIDs).

Most NSAIDs exhibit a spectrum of analgesic, anti-inflammatory, antiplatelet and antipyretic actions, although the degree to which these are seen can vary between different drugs. In general these effects are related to the inhibition of the enzyme cyclo-oxygenase (COX) and therefore to the synthesis of prostaglandins, prostacyclins and thromboxane A_2 from arachidonic acid.

Two types of COX enzyme have been described, COX-1 and COX-2. The former is *constitutive* and is normally present in most body tissues such as the kidney, gastrointestinal mucosa and platelets, where prostaglandin production helps to maintain normal organ function. Inhibition of COX-1 is thought to be responsible for most of the adverse effects of NSAIDs. The second type, COX-2, is *inducible* and produced as a result of inflammation or tissue damage. Inhibition of this enzyme will have mainly analgesic and anti-inflammatory effects. Newer NSAIDs (COX-2 inhibitors), that affect only COX-2, appear to be associated with fewer adverse effects.

While the analgesic actions of NSAIDs have been presumed to result primarily from a peripheral site of action, this may not be the case. There is some evidence that a central mechanism of action augments the peripheral effects. In addition, it is possible that NSAIDs may possess other pharmacological properties and that some of their effects may not be mediated by inhibition of COX.

The NSAIDs are rapidly absorbed from the upper gastrointestinal tract, primarily from the stomach. Peak plasma concentrations are usually reached about 2 hours after oral administration. Most NSAIDs are metabolized in the liver and their metabolites excreted by the kidney. Clearance is reduced in elderly patients and in those with renal disease. Most NSAIDs have half-lives of 2–3 hours although some, like piroxicam and tenoxicam, are much longer (50–60 hours), enabling these drugs to be given just once a day. The NSAIDs with longer half-lives may be associated with a higher incidence of adverse effects.

ANALGESIC EFFECTS

Nonsteroidal anti-inflammatory drugs may be used as the sole method of treatment for mild to moderate pain. They are not sufficiently effective as the sole agent after major surgery or injury in most patients, in whom they are best used in combination with other analgesics such as opioids. They can, however, lead to better analgesia than lower-potency opioids such as codeine and propoxyphene.

When used in combination with opioids NSAIDs may enhance the quality of analgesia. They may also lead to a 20–40% reduction in opioid requirement, although there is no consistent evidence to show that this 'opioid-sparing' effect results in a significant reduction in the incidence of opioid-related side effects. When NSAIDs are used *instead* of opioids, a significant reduction in side effects is seen.

There is a 'ceiling effect' to the analgesia produced by these drugs, when further increases in dose do not result in additional pain relief, but may result in an increase in adverse effects. There appears to be little if any difference in analgesic efficacy between the different NSAIDs, although differences may exist in their anti-inflammatory activity and in the incidence of side effects. While concurrent use of another NSAID is not usually recommended, pain relief can be improved by the addition of acetaminophen (paracetamol).

Most NSAIDs are given orally or rectally. Some (e.g. ketorolac, tenoxicam and diclofenac) can be given by injection. Oral administration is very effective and there is little evidence that other routes offer significant advantages in terms of analgesic efficacy or side effects.

ADVERSE EFFECTS

The NSAIDs can produce a variety of undesirable adverse effects, so the potential risk of using these drugs should always be weighed against possible benefits. The comments below refer to the commonly used NSAIDs that have both COX-1 and COX-2 activity, although the degree of inhibition of each enzyme may vary between drugs.

Gastrointestinal

Reductions in prostaglandin levels may lead to erosions of the gastrointestinal mucosa (especially in the stomach). This is due to a reduction in the prostaglandin-mediated protective functions of mucus production, maintenance of mucosal blood flow, and inhibition of gastric acid secretion. Thus, the problem will not be avoided if the drugs are given by parenteral or rectal routes. The benefit of prophylaxis against gastric effects is unclear.

Prostaglandin analogs (e.g. misoprostol) are possibly more effective that H_2 antagonists (e.g. cimetidine, ranitidine) in reducing the incidence of these side effects.

Gastric irritation, dyspepsia and ulceration (which may be silent in approximately 50% of patients until a bleed or perforation occurs) may develop at any time, but are less likely with short-term treatment. The risk of gastrointestinal side effects increases with increasing age, alcohol, history of peptic ulcer disease and/or gastric bleeding, high doses, and concurrent use of anticoagulants (including heparin used for thromboprophylaxis) or steroids. Ibuprofen appears to have one of the lowest incidences of gastrointestinal side effects; piroxicam is associated with one of the highest.

Renal

In patients in whom the effective circulating blood volume is decreased (e.g. as a result of hypovolemia, dehydration, hypotension, sepsis or excessive use of diuretics) or in patients with congestive cardiac failure or hepatic cirrhosis, vasodilatory renal prostaglandins are released in order to maintain renal perfusion. A reduction in prostaglandin levels due to NSAID administration may result in decreases in renal blood flow and acute renal failure. Pre-existing renal impairment will increase the risk of renal complications. It should be noted that elderly patients often have reduced renal function even though serum creatinine levels appear normal. Concurrent administration of some other drugs may also increase the risk of renal problems with NSAIDs. These include angiotensin-converting enzyme (ACE) inhibitors, potassium-sparing diuretics, methotrexate and cyclosporin.

Acute postoperative renal failure due to NSAIDs has been reported even in healthy young patients. Many perioperative factors may adversely affect renal blood flow and it may be wise, in some cases, to delay administration of NSAIDs until the postoperative period and until the patients is normovolemic and normotensive. If a patient is already receiving an NSAID, it should be discontinued if there is any increase in plasma urea or creatinine, or if urine output is low.

Nonsteroidal anti-inflammatory drugs can cause sodium, potassium and water retention, which may lead to edema in some patients, and may reduce the effectiveness of antihypertensive therapy. Interstitial nephritis and nephrotic syndrome have also been reported in association with NSAID use.

Platelet function and bleeding times

Aggregation of platelets depends on thromboxane A_2. As formation of thromboxane A_2 is reduced by NSAID-induced inhibition of COX, bleeding times may be prolonged. This may increase the risk of perioperative blood loss in some situations, although this effect is not usually clinically significant.

Aspirin is particularly effective in inhibiting platelet function as it *irreversibly* inhibits COX and effectively prolongs bleeding time for the life of the platelet (4–8 days). Recovery depends on the production of new platelets. Other NSAIDs *reversibly* inhibit platelet COX and the effect lasts only as long as the drug remains in the patient.

Respiratory

Bronchospasm, related to COX inhibition, can occur in some asthmatic subjects, and NSAIDs should be used with caution in these patients. Up to 5–10% of adult asthmatic patients may develop aspirin-induced asthma and a cross-sensitivity can exist between aspirin and other NSAIDs.

Other effects

Headache, anxiety, depression, confusion, dizziness and somnolence have all been reported, as have a variety of skin reactions and blood dyscrasias. Abnormalities in liver function tests may occur but are usually transient.

Nonsteroidal anti-inflammatory drugs may affect the actions of other drugs that are dependent on the kidney for excretion, such as the aminoglycoside antibiotics (e.g. gentamicin) and digoxin.

PRECAUTIONS AND CONTRAINDICATIONS

Before NSAIDs are prescribed, reference should be made to the appropriate product information sheet for each drug. Precautions, contraindications, suggested doses and duration of therapy, potential drug interactions and permitted routes of administration may vary between different drugs and different countries.

An evidence-based report by the Royal College of Anaesthetists considered the use of NSAIDs in the postoperative period and suggested certain precautions and contraindications. These are summarized in **Box 7.1**.

ACETAMINOPHEN (PARACETAMOL)

Although acetaminophen is considered by some to be an NSAID, its action is believed to result from inhibition of prostaglandin synthesis within the central nervous system. Acetaminophen is analgesic and antipyretic but has no anti-inflammatory activity. It does not cause gastrointestinal ulceration or bleeding.

Most of the drug is excreted by the kidney after glucuronide and sulfate conjugation in the liver. A small proportion is metabolized to form the potentially hepatotoxic metabolite N-acetyl-p-benzoquinoneimine (NAPQI). This metabolite is normally inactivated by conjugation with hepatic glutathione to produce a nontoxic metabolite that is excreted in the urine. If large amounts of NAPQI are produced following large doses of acetaminophen, hepatic glutathione may be depleted and reaction of NAPQI with hepatic proteins increased. This may lead to hepatic necrosis.

Susceptibility to hepatic toxicity is said to be increased in patients with chronic alcoholism. Therapeutic ingestion of acetaminophen is reported to be a common cause of acute liver failure in these patients. The mechanism for this remains unclear but reasons may include decreased hepatic levels of glutathione and/or higher levels of NAPQI. Susceptibility may also be increased in patients with chronic liver disease.

Side effects of the drug are normally minimal. It is generally recommended that doses do not exceed 4 g per day in adults, but

Possible precautions and contraindications to the use of NSAIDs for acute pain management

NSAIDs should be avoided in the following clinical situations:
- pre-existing renal impairment (elevated plasma creatinine levels)
- hyperkalemia
- dehydration, hypovolemia or hypotension from any cause
- cardiac failure
- severe liver dysfunction
- uncontrolled hypertension
- aspirin-induced asthma
- history of gastrointestinal bleeding or ulceration
- known hypersensitivity to aspirin or other NSAIDs

NSAIDs should be used with caution in the following clinical situations:
- impaired hepatic function, diabetes, bleeding or coagulation disorders, vascular disease
- operations where there is a high risk of intraoperative hemorrhage (e.g. cardiac, major vascular and hepatobiliary surgery)
- operations where an absence of bleeding is important (e.g. eye surgery, neurosurgery and cosmetic surgery)
- other forms of asthma
- concurrent use of other NSAIDs (except acetaminophen), ACE inhibitors, potassium-sparing diuretics, anticoagulants, methotrexate, cyclosporin and antibiotics such as gentamicin
- children less than 16 years old
- pregnant and lactating women
- advanced age (renal impairment is likely in patients older than 65 years, even if creatinine levels are normal)

Box 7.1

Many perioperative factors may adversely affect renal blood flow and it may be wise to delay administration of NSAIDs until the postoperative period and until the patient is normovolemic and normotensive. If a patient is already receiving an NSAID, it should be discontinued if there is any increase in plasma urea or creatinine levels, or if urine output is low. Adapted from the guidelines of the Royal College of Anaesthetists (1998).

it may be reasonable to allow up to 6 g per day for 3–4 days in some patients after surgery or injury.

Acetaminophen is usually given by oral or rectal routes. After oral administration and absorption from the small bowel, peak plasma concentrations are reached within about an hour. An intravenous preparation, *propacetamol*, has been released in some countries. This is a 'prodrug' which is rapidly hydrolyzed by plasma esterases to acetaminophen.

NMDA RECEPTOR ANTAGONIST DRUGS

Tissue damage or inflammation, occurring after surgery or trauma, causes pain stimuli to be carried along peripheral sensory nerves to the spinal cord. Persistent input of pain stimuli from the site of injury leads to changes in the way in which spinal cord neurons process the information received from the periphery.

Repetitive input of painful stimuli can lead to the development of spinal cord neuron hyperexcitability, and an increased sensitivity and exaggerated response to further pain stimuli (*hyperalgesia*). The increased sensitivity may also be to stimuli that would not normally be regarded as painful (e.g. touch), but because of these changes result in the sensation of pain (*allodynia*). This phenomenon of hyperexcitability is referred to as *central sensitization*. It may lead to alterations in the nature of the pain perceived or increases in its intensity and duration. *Wind-up* refers to a phenomenon in which spinal cord neurons show a progressively greater response to repetitive but constant intensity stimuli. Wind-up and central sensitization are not identical processes but it is likely that events resembling wind-up underlie the development of central sensitization. In most patients after an acute injury, central sensitization appears to be reversed as the injury heals and acute pain resolves. In some patients, however, the condition becomes chronic.

It is thought that *N*-methyl-D-aspartate (NMDA) receptors, located in the spinal cord, are involved in the development of wind-up and central sensitization. There is evidence for NMDA receptor involvement in many types of pain – inflammatory, postoperative, neuropathic and ischemic. Drugs that act as antagonists at these receptors may not only prevent the development of wind-up and central sensitization, but may also downregulate hyperexcitability after sensitization has taken place. The use of NMDA receptor antagonist drugs is increasingly common in the management of acute and chronic pain states.

The NMDA receptor antagonist drugs have been used in a number of clinical situations (**Box 7.2**). In acute pain management, they are usually administered as an adjunct to local anaesthetic drugs, opioids or other analgesic agents. In this situation they may improve the quality of pain relief, reduce the amount of opioid needed for analgesia, and lead to a reduction in opioid-related side effects. Whether or not their use can reliably prevent subsequent chronic pain syndromes (such as post-thoracotomy, post-mastectomy and phantom pain) is still unknown, although initial results are promising. These drugs have been shown to be effective in the treatment of neuropathic pain (see Chapter 10).

The NMDA receptor may also have a role in the development of tolerance, and NMDA receptor antagonists may block, and even reverse, morphine tolerance and dependence.

KETAMINE

The most common NMDA receptor antagonist in clinical use is ketamine, which is a drug that has been used as an anesthetic agent for many years. It is most commonly available as a racemic

---

Possible uses for NMDA receptor antagonist drugs

- treatment of acute pain
- prevention (? reversal) of central sensitization and wind-up
- management of neuropathic pain
- management of pain in opioid-tolerant patients

Box 7.2

mixture of R and S isomers. The S isomer, available in some countries only, is a more potent analgesic and produces fewer side effects than the R isomer. Ketamine acts at a number of receptors including NMDA and opioid receptors, although interactions at receptors other than the NMDA receptor appear to be of limited clinical importance.

The terminal elimination half-life of ketamine is 2–3 hours. The drug is metabolized by the liver and the metabolites are excreted by the kidney. The primary metabolite, norketamine, is less potent than ketamine but may contribute to its analgesic action.

When used in pain management, ketamine is usually administered by intravenous (IV) or subcutaneous (SC) routes. It should only be prescribed by those who are familiar with the drug.

Analgesic activity

In contrast to other anesthetic agents, ketamine can provide excellent analgesia when given in subanesthetic doses. The NMDA receptor and opioid-sparing effects of ketamine may be seen with infusion rates as low as 1 µg/kg per minute (about 100 mg per day in an average adult), especially if a small loading dose (e.g. 100–200 µg/kg) is given prior to the start of the infusion.

In some centers, ketamine is added to the opioid used in patient-controlled analgesia, so that the patient receives both opioid and ketamine with every demand. However, large interpatient variations in opioid requirements mean that patients are likely to receive widely varying doses of ketamine. This could lead to inadequate therapy in some patients and an increased risk of adverse effects in others.

Side effects

One of the main problems with ketamine is that it interferes with sensory perception as well as the perception of pain. As a result, its use has been associated with psychotomimetic side effects. With higher doses these effects include dreaming (pleasant or unpleasant), hallucinations, and emergence (from anesthesia) excitation, agitation and delirium. These side effects may be reduced by the concurrent administration of benzodiazepines.

In the smaller doses commonly used as an adjunct to other analgesics, side effects may still occur (albeit infrequently) and may include dizziness and feelings of unreality or 'floating'. To a large extent these effects are dose-related and are probably negligible at doses of 1–2 µg/kg per minute. In these low doses, significant cardiovascular or respiratory effects have not been reported.

DEXTROMETHORPHAN

Dextromethorphan is widely available as an over-the-counter cough suppressant. It is not in common clinical use.

ALPHA-2-ADRENERGIC AGONIST DRUGS

Alpha-2 adrenoreceptors (or α_2 receptors) are located on peripheral sensory nerve terminals and in the spinal cord and brain stem. The receptors in the spinal cord are thought to be primarily responsible for the analgesic effects of α_2-adrenergic agonist drugs such as clonidine. These drugs are normally used in combination with other analgesic drugs such as local anesthetics or opioids.

CLONIDINE

Clonidine is the α_2 agonist most commonly used in clinical practice. It is available in tablet or injectable form – the latter for parenteral injection (IV, SC or intramuscular) or addition to solutions used in regional anesthesia or analgesia (including epidural and intrathecal analgesia). A transdermal patch is also available. Approximately 50% of clonidine is metabolized in the liver, the remaining drug being excreted unchanged by the kidney.

Introduced initially as a nasal decongestant and used as an antihypertensive for years, clonidine is also an effective analgesic. By itself it has been used for pain relief after a variety of surgical procedures, although it is normally used in combination with other analgesic drugs. In acute pain management, combination with opioid analgesia can lead to improved pain relief and a reduction in opioid requirements. Added to solutions used for epidural, intrathecal and other major regional (e.g. brachial or lumbar plexus) anesthesia and analgesia, clonidine has been shown to increase the duration of pain relief. In general, administration by epidural and intrathecal routes is more effective than IV or oral administration.

The routine use of clonidine in acute pain management has been limited by side effects, particularly hypotension and sedation. Other possible side effects include bradycardia, dizziness, dry mouth, decreased bowel motility, and diuresis.

Clonidine may be effective in the treatment of neuropathic pain and other forms of chronic and cancer pain. It has also been used in the management of withdrawal from opioids, benzodiazepines and alcohol. Abrupt cessation of clonidine after long-term treatment can itself lead to a withdrawal syndrome, the signs and symptoms of which can include restlessness, headache, nausea, insomnia, rebound hypertension and cardiac arrhythmias.

DEXMEDETOMIDINE
Dexmedetomidine is a more specific and shorter-acting α_2 agonist. It is mainly used in clinical studies.

NITROUS OXIDE

Nitrous oxide is commonly used in some countries as a combination of 50% nitrous oxide and 50% oxygen in premixed cylinders (Entonox). In other countries, the use of a mixing valve permits a variety of nitrous oxide/oxygen combinations to be used. A one-way demand valve allows delivery of the gas when the patient inspires, providing there is an airtight fit between face and mask or mouthpiece. The technique is inherently safe as it is self-administered. If the patient becomes too drowsy the mask will fall away from the patient's face.

The onset of analgesia is rapid and some effect will be seen after four or five deep breaths. Offset of effect is also rapid so analgesia can only be maintained by repeated inhalations. For this reason nitrous oxide is usually only ordered for short painful procedures, such as coughing and breathing exercises in patients with fractured ribs, removal of drains, or dressing changes. It will normally be used in combination with opioid or other analgesic therapies. In some institutions, concerns about environmental nitrous oxide levels limit the use of nitrous oxide in general wards.

POSSIBLE COMPLICATIONS AND CONTRAINDICATIONS

Air-containing spaces

Nitrous oxide is contraindicated in the presence of air-containing spaces such as a pneumothorax or intracranial air. Gases equilibrate across permeable membranes so that concentrations on either side become equal. Nitrous oxide equilibrates rapidly; nitrogen much more slowly. If a patient breathes a mixture containing only oxygen and nitrous oxide, the concentration of nitrous oxide in any air-containing space will rise rapidly. However, the concentration of nitrogen in that space will fall much more slowly so that there is an overall increase in volume of the gas space. If the space cannot expand there can be a marked increase in pressure.

Inactivation of vitamin B_{12}

Nitrous oxide oxidizes vitamin B_{12}, changing it from an active to an inactive form. Oxidation of vitamin B_{12} in turn inactivates the enzyme methionine synthetase, which leads to decreased formation of methionine and tetrahydrofolate (THF). This inactivation appears to be irreversible and may apply to stores of vitamin B_{12} as well as vitamin B_{12} bound to methionine synthetase.

Methionine is required for normal myelination and a lack of methionine may lead to demyelination of nerves and consequent neurological signs and symptoms. Tetrahydrofolate is required for the synthesis of deoxythymidine, which is essential for normal DNA production. If THF formation is decreased, changes are likely to be seen in cells with a rapid turnover, such as occurs in the bone marrow. This can lead to megaloblastic bone marrow changes and agranulocytosis.

Clinical features of nitrous oxide-induced inactivation of vitamin B_{12}

Both hematologic and neurologic complications have been reported following prolonged or repeated administration of nitrous oxide. The exact duration of exposure required to cause these changes is unknown. The clinical features resemble those of vitamin B_{12} deficiency. However, vitamin B_{12} levels may be normal, as the problem is due to a reduction in *active* vitamin B_{12} levels, not necessarily total body levels.

Megaloblastic changes in bone marrow may lead to red blood cells that are larger than normal. The patient may also be anemic. These changes may be more likely in patients with significant other illnesses.

Neurologic consequences of nitrous oxide administration appear to be much less common, and much less well recognized, than hematologic changes. They seem to occur mainly in one of two circumstances: the abuse of nitrous oxide, or where there is a pre-existing vitamin B_{12} deficiency (clinical or subclinical). In the latter group neurologic signs and symptoms have been reported after a single anesthetic use of nitrous oxide.

Treatment or prevention of nitrous oxide-induced inactivation of vitamin B_{12}

There is a paucity of evidence relating to prevention or treatment of complications due to nitrous oxide-related inactivation of vitamin B_{12}. As nitrous oxide interferes with the function of vitamin B_{12}, it is possible that vitamin B_{12} supplements may not help unless given at a time remote from the administration of nitrous oxide (difficult when repeat administration is occurring). There is no clear support in the literature for the use of vitamin B_{12} supplements in this situation. Methionine supplements have been suggested for the prevention of neurologic changes, but evidence for their benefit is limited. Some evidence exists for the role of folinic acid (5-formyl-THF) in preventing or reversing nitrous oxide-induced bone marrow changes.

REFERENCES AND FURTHER READING

Dickenson A.H. (1995) Spinal cord pharmacology of pain. *British Journal of Anaesthesia* **75**, 169–176.

Eisenach J.C., De Kock M. and Klimscha W. (1995) α_2-adrenergic agonists for regional anesthesia: a clinical review of clonidine. *Anesthesiology* **85**, 655–674.

Gould T.H., Cockings J.G.L. and Buist M. (1997) Postoperative acute liver failure after therapeutic paracetamol administration. *Anaesthesia and Intensive Care* **25**, 153–155.

Khan Z.P., Ferguson C.N. and Jones R.M. (1999) Alpha-2 and imidazoline receptor agonists: their pharmacology and therapeutic role. *Anaesthesia* **54**, 146–165.

Kohrs R. and Durieux M.E. (1998) Ketamine: teaching an old drug new tricks. *Anesthesia and Analgesia* **87**, 1186–1193.

Nunn J.F. (1987) Clinical aspects of the interaction between nitrous oxide and vitamin B_{12}. *British Journal of Anaesthesia* **59**, 3–13.

Royal College of Anaesthetists (1998) *Guidelines for the use of non-steroidal anti-inflammatory drugs in the perioperative period*. London: Royal College of Anaesthetists.

Schmid R.L., Sandler A.N. and Katz J. (1999) Use and efficacy of low-dose ketamine in the management of acute postoperative pain: a review of current techniques and outcomes. *Pain* **82**, 111–125.

Tarkkila P. and Rosenbery P.H. (1998) Perioperative analgesia with non-steroidal analgesics. *Current Opinion in Anaesthesiology* **11**, 407–410.

Wiebalck C.A. and Van Aken H. (1995) Paracetamol and propacetamol for postoperative pain: contrasts to traditional NSAIDs. *Baillière's Clinical Anaesthesiology* **9**, 469–481.

Woolf C.J. (1995) Somatic pain – pathogenesis and prevention. *British Journal of Anaesthesia* **75**, 169–176.

CHAPTER 8

OTHER TECHNIQUES IN ACUTE PAIN MANAGEMENT

Continuous regional neural blockade

Nonpharmacologic therapies

There are a number of additional techniques that can be used in the management of acute pain, either alone or in combination with other methods of analgesia. These include other pharmacologic therapies as well as nonpharmacologic treatments.

CONTINUOUS REGIONAL NEURAL BLOCKADE

The use of local anesthesia in the performance of 'single-shot' regional neural blockade (one-time nerve or nerve plexus block) is common practice in anesthesia. While this may provide many hours of analgesia after surgery, an alternative technique will be required if pain relief is to be continued further into the postoperative period. The benefits of 'single-shot' blockade can be sustained for a number of days if a catheter is placed at the time of nerve or plexus block. This allows local anesthetic drugs to be given either by repeated bolus dose or by continuous infusion.

Compared with continuous epidural analgesia, continuous regional neural blockade may have advantages in certain situations. For example, patients with an abnormality in their coagulation status may be at risk of a spinal hematoma following placement of an epidural needle or catheter. As outlined in Chapter 6, this could have devastating neurologic consequences. In such patients, the use of a continuous regional analgesic technique may be a much safer alternative.

Continuous regional neural blockade will normally be initiated and managed by anesthesiologists. Standard orders and nursing policies and procedures are recommended and all catheters should carry a clearly visible label.

CONTINUOUS UPPER OR LOWER LIMB REGIONAL ANALGESIA

A catheter placed near the brachial plexus (by any of the usual approaches) can be used for continuous brachial plexus analgesia. This may be used for pain relief following most types of upper limb surgery or injury (e.g. traumatic amputation). In addition to pain relief, the sympathetic blockade that results can be beneficial in situations where vasodilatation of blood vessels in the arm is required (e.g. after microvascular surgery).

In the lower limb, continuous femoral nerve, 'three-in-one' (femoral, obturator and lateral femoral cutaneous nerves) and lumbar plexus blocks can give excellent analgesia following surgery. Catheters may also be placed close to the sciatic or posterior tibial nerves, and adjacent to, or directly into, the sheath of a transected nerve following limb amputation (e.g. the sciatic nerve following lower limb amputation).

A 'single-shot' femoral nerve block can provide rapid pain relief in patients who have sustained a fractured femur. It helps to reduce spasm of the quadriceps muscle, which inevitably accompanies this fracture and exacerbates the pain. It is well worth instituting before the patient is moved, for instance from the emergency department trolley to the operating table.

Maintenance of analgesia

As is the case with epidural analgesia in the postoperative period, the aim will usually be to provide good pain relief (and, possibly sympathetic blockade) without significant motor block. This allows motor function to be monitored and physiotherapy (where indicated) to be carried out.

The degree of block produced will depend on the dose of local anesthetic drug given – the lower the total dose, the less the chance of significant motor blockade. Examples of solutions commonly used for infusion are 0.125% bupivacaine or 0.2%

ropivacaine. In some situations higher concentrations may be necessary.

NONPHARMACOLOGIC THERAPIES

Nonpharmacologic therapies (**Box 8.1**) can also be used in the treatment of acute pain and may be beneficial for some patients. Alone, these strategies will usually not be effective for the treatment of moderate to severe acute pain. They should therefore be considered as supplementary to the pharmacologic or invasive techniques described in earlier chapters.

COGNITIVE-BEHAVIORAL INTERVENTIONS

According to cognitive-behavioral theory, pain is a complex sensory and emotional experience. That is, the intensity of acute pain perceived and the patient's response to pain and pain therapy may be influenced by a number of psychological, behavioral, environmental, social and physical factors. For example, anxiety and fear, which commonly accompany acute pain, have been shown to increase the amount of pain perceived, analgesic requirements and the tendency to report normally

Examples of nonpharmacologic interventions

Cognitive-behavioral	Physical
Reassurance	Applications of heat and cold
Education/information	Massage, exercise and immobilization
Relaxation	Transcutaneous electrical nerve stimulation (TENS)
Imagery	Acupuncture
Distraction	
Behavioral instruction	
Hypnosis	

Box 8.1

Adapted from Carr et al. (1992).

nonpainful stimulation as pain. Highly aggressive and angry patients also tend to require higher doses of analgesics. Depression has been associated with higher pain ratings but is a less common response to acute pain. The meaning that a person attaches to pain can also influence perception of pain intensity and the ability to tolerate pain. For example, perceived pain may be different if an operation for cancer is curative compared with an operation that is palliative only.

Locus of control testing may show how patients will respond and adapt to surgical pain. Those with an 'internal' locus of control believe that they can, through their own behavior, exert control over their health. A perception of lack of control in this group increases anxiety. Those with an 'external' locus of control believe that what they do will have little or no influence on the outcome of their health and that their health is in the hands of fate, chance or other people. This latter group may be very dependent on the ward staff, may report high pain scores despite appearing fairly comfortable, and may not manage well with techniques such as PCA. It is possible that up to 20% of patients find the responsibility for control stress-inducing.

Coping styles may also affect self-reports of pain and the ability to tolerate pain. Occasional discrepancies between pain behavior and a patient's self-report of pain may result from different coping skills. Staff should not necessarily assume, for example, that a patient who is smiling, reading or sleeping is comfortable.

Cognitive-behavioral therapies (including those listed in **Box 8.1**) are derived from the study of learning and behavior change. They can be used to alter the way in which patients perceive, interpret and react to pain. They aim to help patients understand more about their pain, take an active part in pain assessment and control, alter their behavior in response to pain and improve their coping skills.

Education and information about expected discomfort, ways to decrease pain and details of all procedures (see Chapter 12) can decrease anxiety, analgesic use and self-reports of pain. Similar reductions may also follow the use of simple relaxation strategies (e.g. controlled breathing, muscle relaxation), distraction (e.g. music) and imagery (e.g. imagining pleasant

Transc

Although g…
be useful in r…
reports of pain afte…
in some patients. It may …
pain (see Chapter 10). It is no…
other pain relief therapies and not as th…
for acute pain.

The technique is simple, safe, noninvasive, free from systemic side effects and allows patients some control over their own therapy. The battery-powered TENS unit generates a small electric current which is transmitted to electrodes placed on the skin. The best effect is achieved when the electrodes are placed over the affected dermatomes or over acupuncture points. The amplitude and frequency of the current delivered are varied by the patient according to the severity of the pain. The current is altered so that it is at an intensity low enough to produce only a comfortable buzzing or tingling on the skin. Both high-frequency (e.g. 100 Hz) and low-frequency (e.g. 2–4 Hz) currents have been used with TENS. It is possible that better results are obtained by using a mixed mode (i.e. an alternating pattern of high and low frequencies).

The analgesic effects of TENS are thought to result, at least in part, from the release of endogenous opioids.

Pub.

h, Public

...tion is important in
...utaneous electrical nerve
...nal of Anaesthesia **77**, 798–803.

...H.J. et al. (1997) The influence of
...ative anxiety and physical complaints in patients
...gery. Pain **69**, 19–25.

Ferrell B.R. (1996) Patient education and non-drug interventions. In *Pain in the Elderly* (eds Ferrell B.R. and Ferrell B.A.). IASP Task Force on Pain in the Elderly. IASP Publications, Seattle.

Ganapathy S., Wasserman R.A., Watson J.T. et al. (1999) Modified continuous femoral three-in-one block for postoperative pain after total knee arthroplasty. *Anesthesia and Analgesia* **89**, 1197–1202.

Keefe F.J., Beaupré P.M., Weiner D.K. and Siegler I. (1996) Pain in older adults: a cognitive-behavioral perspective. In *Pain in the Elderly* (eds Ferrell B.R. and Ferrell B.A.). IASP Task Force on Pain in the Elderly. IASP Publications, Seattle.

McKenzie A.G. and Mathe S. (1996) Interpleural local anaesthesia: anatomical basis for mechanism of action. *British Journal of Anaesthesia* **76**, 297–299.

National Health and Medical Research Council (1999) *Acute Pain Management: The Scientific Evidence.* Canberra (available at http://www.nhmrc.health.gov.au/publicat/pdf/cp57.pdf).

Pettersson N., Perbeck L., Brismar B. and Hahn R.G. (1997) Sensory and sympathetic block during interpleural analgesia. *Regional Anesthesia* **22**, 313–317.

Thomas V., Heath M., Rose D. and Flory P. (1995) Psychological characteristics and the effectiveness of patient-controlled analgesia. *British Journal of Anaesthesia* **74**, 271–276.

CHAPTER 9

THE OPIOID-DEPENDENT PATIENT

Opioid tolerance, dependence and addiction

Categories of opioid-dependent patient

Aims of treatment

Specific analgesic techniques

In earlier chapters emphasis has been placed on the large interpatient variation in the amount of opioid required for effective analgesia and the need to titrate opioid dose to effect for each patient. When patients have been taking opioids for a prolonged period (whether legally prescribed or illegally obtained) effective titration can be much more difficult. Many of these patients will be tolerant to and physically dependent on these drugs; some will have an opioid addiction. It must be emphasized that tolerance and dependence are natural biological consequences of repeated drug use and do *not* imply abuse or addiction.

Provision of effective pain relief in these patients can be a difficult and challenging task and may require significant deviation from standardized protocols. It is recommended that advice regarding analgesia in these patients should be obtained from pain management physicians and other specialists in the relevant areas.

OPIOID TOLERANCE, DEPENDENCE AND ADDICTION

TOLERANCE

Patients on long-term opioid therapy may develop a tolerance to the drug. This term is defined in **Box 9.1.** It refers to the

Tolerance, dependence and addiction

Tolerance	A decrease in sensitivity to opioids resulting in less effect from the same dose, or the need for progressively larger doses to maintain the same effect
Physical dependence	A physiological adaptation to a drug characterized by the emergence of a withdrawal (abstinence) syndrome if the drug is abruptly stopped, reduced in dose, or antagonized
Addiction	A pattern of drug use characterized by aberrant drug-taking behaviors and the compulsive use of a substance in order to experience its psychic effects, or to avoid the effects of its absence (withdrawal). There is continued use despite the risk of physical, psychological or social harm to the user
Pseudoaddiction	Drug-seeking behavior caused by a need for better pain relief

Box 9.1

progressive decrease in effect seen for the same dose of opioid, or the need for progressively larger doses to maintain the same effect. Tolerance develops to analgesia and opioid-related side effects, but to varying degrees and at varying rates.

Tolerance to analgesia

The mechanisms that lead to tolerance are complex and have yet to be fully explained. They are thought to include involvement of the *N*-methyl-D-aspartate (NMDA) receptor. The NMDA receptor antagonist drugs, such as ketamine (see Chapter 7), have been used to block or reverse the development of tolerance to morphine. Tolerance can occur very quickly; it is possible that it develops more rapidly to the highly lipid-soluble opioids such as fentanyl.

In the clinical setting, many patients on long-term opioid therapy will not require dose increases for weeks, months or even years. If dose escalation is evident, causes other than tolerance should also be considered. These include:

- increasing pain due to disease progression (more likely in patients with cancer pain, e.g. due to tumor growth)
- pain due to postoperative complications (e.g. compartment syndrome, peritonitis)
- onset of neuropathic pain (see Chapter 10)
- major psychological distress (e.g. anxiety, depression)
- aberrant drug-taking behaviors (see below)

The practical significance of opioid tolerance in acute pain management is that tolerant patients may require much higher doses of opioid than an opioid-naive patient after a similar injury or operation. Dose regimens therefore need careful titration if effective pain relief is to be achieved. Patient-controlled analgesia (PCA) may be a practical way of allowing the patient to self-titrate these doses (see below).

In a study comparing postoperative opioid-tolerant patients with patients who were opioid-naive (Rapp et al., 1995), pain relief using PCA was noted to be less effective in the former group, despite their much greater opioid requirements.

Tolerance to side effects

Tolerance to the different side effects of opioids develops at different rates. Tolerance to nausea and vomiting, cognitive impairment, sedation and respiratory depression occurs rapidly; tolerance to constipation and miosis develops very slowly, if at all.

Despite tolerance to the effects of opioids, side effects, including respiratory depression, can occur in opioid-tolerant patients if doses are suddenly and markedly increased, as might occur after surgery. In the study by Rapp and coworkers, opioid-tolerant patients using PCA had a much higher incidence of sedation compared with patients who were not opioid-tolerant (Rapp et al., 1995).

Incomplete cross-tolerance

Patients tolerant to one opioid will usually be tolerant to all other opioids. This is called cross-tolerance. However, the degree of cross-tolerance that occurs is unpredictable and appears to be incomplete. If a change is made from one opioid to another, especially when dose requirements have been high, it may be best to commence the new opioid at a dose that is about 50% of the calculated equianalgesic dose of the first drug. Subsequent doses of the alternative opioid should then be titrated to effect.

If a decision is made to change opioid therapy to methadone, doses that are about 10–15% of the expected equianalgesic dose may be more appropriate. The much lower dose required may be due to a number of factors including the long and variable half-life of methadone and its NMDA receptor antagonist properties.

As noted in Chapter 2, equianalgesic doses are based on single-dose studies in opioid-naive patients. The equianalgesic doses of opioids in patients on long-term opioid therapy are unknown and equianalgesic dose tables must be used with caution.

Opioid rotation

If pain is uncontrolled, the first step is usually to increase the dose of opioid. In some patients, especially those requiring high doses, further increases may be limited by intolerable side effects (despite aggressive treatment of the side effects) even though pain relief remains inadequate.

The concept of opioid rotation is still controversial but it refers to the changing from one opioid to another in order to obtain better pain relief and fewer side effects. It is based on the belief that this change will allow clearance of the first opioid and its metabolites, and also takes advantage of the fact that incomplete cross-tolerance is likely to exist.

Although opioid rotation is practiced more frequently in chronic pain settings and especially in palliative care, it may occasionally have a role in acute pain management. An opioid-dependent patient who is requiring high doses of an opioid prior to surgery is likely to need much higher doses in the postoperative period. Therefore, it may be worth considering the use of an alternative opioid in the immediate few days after surgery, especially if inadequate analgesia and/or side effects are seen with increased doses of the original opioid. The alternative opioid may be effective in doses that are much lower than expected (based on equianalgesic doses) because of incomplete cross-tolerance.

If a patient requires high doses of morphine prior to surgery, high levels of morphine metabolites may already be present. Increased dose requirements in the immediate postoperative period will lead to further increases in metabolite levels and metabolite-related side effects (including μ receptor, antalgesic and neuroexcitatory effects – see Chapter 2) may then occur. In this case the use of an alternative opioid after surgery would allow time for clearance of these metabolites.

PHYSICAL DEPENDENCE

Physical dependence refers to the physiological adaptation to opioids, characterized by the development of a withdrawal (or abstinence) syndrome if the opioid is antagonized (by opioid antagonists or agonist-antagonists), suddenly stopped, or abruptly reduced in dose. In other words, continued opioid use is required in order to suppress signs and symptoms of withdrawal.

The lowest dose of an opioid and the shortest duration of treatment that may lead to physical dependence are not known. Dependence should be presumed to exist if repeated doses of an opioid are given over 1–2 weeks. However, the degree of withdrawal that would be experienced if the opioid were abruptly stopped would depend on the doses that had been used.

In acute pain management, development of dependence is usually relatively unimportant. Most patients after surgery or trauma, even if opioids have been required for more than a week or two, tend to reduce their opioid intake as pain becomes less. That is, weaning from opioids occurs naturally and in the majority of patients planned dose reductions are not required.

However, situations can arise in acute pain management when high doses of opioids are abruptly stopped or reduced. For example, a patient on long-term opioid therapy may be given epidural or intrathecal analgesia in the postoperative period. In most cases the amount of opioid delivered by these routes is relatively small and less than that required to prevent the onset of a withdrawal syndrome. Additional systemic opioids may be required.

Another example is a patient who requires high doses of opioid several days after surgery, but is otherwise ready for discharge from hospital. In this situation, a discharge prescription may be necessary for the purpose of tapering the opioid dose, in order to prevent a withdrawal syndrome after the patient has returned home. Liaison with the patient's family practitioner may be advisable.

Withdrawal (abstinence) syndrome

Signs and symptoms of withdrawal syndrome include yawning, sweating, lacrimation, rhinorrhea, anxiety, restlessness, insomnia, dilated pupils, piloerection, chills, tachycardia, hypertension, nausea and vomiting, crampy abdominal pains, diarrhea, and muscle aches and pains. Piloerection results in the appearance of gooseflesh so that the skin resembles that of a plucked turkey. Thus the expression 'going cold turkey' is used to describe the syndrome of abrupt withdrawal from opioids.

In patients dependent on short-acting opioids, withdrawal may occur as soon as 4–6 hours after the last dose. The prevention of withdrawal syndrome is discussed later in this chapter.

ADDICTION

A major concern for both staff and patients is the fear of addiction (also called 'substance dependence') to opioids given to relieve pain. This has led to undertreatment of pain in many instances. In reality, the risk of addiction from opioids taken to relieve acute pain is very small. In 11 882 inpatients given at least one opioid preparation, Porter and Jick (1980) reported only four documented cases of addiction in patients with no prior history of substance abuse – an incidence of 0.03%. It has been said that those who prescribe and administer the opioids are more at risk of addiction than the patients receiving them.

Addiction requires more than just exposure to a potentially addictive drug. Variables such as peer or family pressures, personality disorders, genetic predisposition and mental, physical and economic distress, may all play a part.

Patients who are addicted to opioids may also be tolerant to their effects and may be physically dependent on the drugs, although this need not be the case. It is their aberrant drug-taking behavioral patterns and loss of personal control that distinguish them from other patients on long-term opioid therapy. There is a physical and psychological need for the drug. Compulsive use of that drug occurs despite the risk of physical, psychological or social harm. Commonly, such patients are willing to acquire the drug by deception or by illegal means.

Aberrant drug-taking behaviors

A wide variety of aberrant drug-taking behaviors have been described, some of which are said to be less common but more suggestive of addiction (**Box 9.2**); others more common but less suggestive of addiction (**Box 9.3**). The latter are more likely to reflect undertreated distress of some kind (e.g. pain or psychological distress). Patients who are anxious, depressed or who have borderline personality disorders, may exhibit some aberrant drug-taking behaviors.

Pseudoaddiction

Occasionally, staff may report that a patient is 'becoming addicted' to opioids when the patient appears to be demanding pain-relieving drugs and exhibiting aberrant drug-taking

Drug-taking behaviors that may be suggestive of addiction

- polysubstance use/abuse (e.g. alcohol, sedatives)
- seeking drugs from other medical sources (e.g. forging or altering prescriptions, 'doctor shopping', 'lost' prescriptions)
- seeking drugs from nonmedical sources (e.g. stealing, borrowing, illegal sources of medical or illicit drugs)
- multiple unsanctioned dose escalations or other noncompliance with treatment
- deteriorating ability to function at work or socially
- diversion of drugs (e.g. selling the drugs)
- injection of oral preparations of a drug (e.g. methadone syrup)

Box 9.2
Adapted from Passik and Portenoy (1998).

Drug-taking behaviors that are less suggestive of addiction

- one or two unsanctioned dose escalations or other noncompliance with treatment
- use of the drug to treat other symptoms
- complaints (sometimes aggressive) about the need for higher doses
- attempts to negotiate treatment
- requesting or demanding specific drugs
- hoarding drugs

Box 9.3
Adapted from Passik and Portenoy (1998).

behaviors similar to those seen in patients with an opioid addiction. However, patients may seek or demand more analgesia if pain relief is inadequate. Undertreatment of acute pain may lead to iatrogenic drug-seeking behaviors that are really pain-avoidance behaviors. This has been termed *pseudoaddiction* by Weisman and Haddox (1989).

CATEGORIES OF OPIOID-DEPENDENT PATIENT

Opioid-dependent patients are often divided into three groups:
- those with cancer pain
- those with chronic noncancer pain
- those with a past or current addiction to opioids

In the acute pain management setting, this grouping of patients is not necessarily helpful. Some staff may even 'rate' patients according to group, ranging from those 'worthy of good treatment' to those 'not so worthy'. They may also have preconceived ideas about who will be a 'good' patient and easy to treat, and who are likely to be 'difficult and demanding'. These attitudes are to be strongly discouraged.

'Difficult' personalities can certainly add to the challenges of treatment, but patients may be much less 'difficult' if they perceive that staff are taking their pain reports and pain management seriously.

From a practical point of view, patients in all three groups are likely to be tolerant to and have a physical dependence on opioids. What can make effective pain management more difficult is whether these patients exhibit, or have exhibited, any aberrant drug-taking behaviors. Although these behaviors are more likely to be seen in patients with an addiction to opioids, they may be seen in some patients on long-term opioid therapy for chronic noncancer pain, and much less commonly in patients with cancer. Particularly challenging for the treating physician is the patient with chronic pain, who shows significant aberrant drug-taking behaviors, and who then has an operation or accident resulting in acute pain.

AIMS OF TREATMENT

The principles of acute pain management in the opioid-dependent patient are similar regardless of the group to which the patient belongs. The main differences in treatment occur when the patient also exhibits some of the aberrant drug-taking behaviors described above.

The aims of treatment (**Box 9.4**) are to bring acute pain (the 'new' pain) under control as effectively and quickly as possible. A

Aims of treatment

- provision of analgesia
- prevention of withdrawal
- management of withdrawal from other drugs
- involvement of multidisciplinary and/or other specialist teams and treatment of comorbidities (depression, etc.) as needed
- management of aberrant drug-taking behaviors

Box 9.4

patient who has a concurrent chronic pain problem (e.g. back pain) needs to be aware that the main aim of treatment, in the first instance at least, is to manage the acute episode.

As opioids will frequently be used in the treatment of acute pain in opioid-dependent patients, most of the following discussion centers on this group of drugs. Before they are administered, the amount of opioid the patient has been taking prior to admission may need to be confirmed with the prescriber.

ANALGESIA

Well-established guidelines for acute pain management provide a useful framework for analgesic use in opioid-tolerant patients, as they do for those who are opioid-naive.

Preferred opioid

Pure opioid agonists are usually the drugs of choice at this time, as there is no ceiling to the dose that can be given in the absence of side effects. The exception is meperidine (pethidine), where doses should be limited because of potential problems with normeperidine toxicity (see Chapter 2). Generally, meperidine is best avoided in these patients.

In general, opioids with a rapid onset of action are abused more commonly than those with a slower onset of effect. Although lipid solubility of the drug plays a role in rate of onset, route of administration and dose may be more important in clinical acute pain management. While controlled-release or long-acting drugs may be preferred for long-term therapy, immediate-release opioids are usually needed for the management of pain in the immediate postoperative or post-injury period, as they allow greater flexibility and more rapid titration.

Using an opioid other than the one the patient is using long-term (opioid rotation) may be an advantage in some circumstances.

Dosages of opioid

Opioid requirements will often be much higher than 'average' in the immediate period after surgery or major injury. The amount of opioid needed can be difficult to judge. It may be best to start with a conservative estimate and then rapidly titrate the drug until the patient is comfortable (based on assessment criteria including function). The dose prescribed should take into account the patient's current opioid requirement, although these estimates may be difficult to obtain when illicit drugs have been used. In the short term and in the absence of any contraindication, the total dose may be increased until satisfactory analgesia is obtained or until side effects limit further increases.

The patient should be assured that staff will aim for good analgesia. However, safety is paramount and the onset of sedation or other significant side effects may prevent further dose escalation. In the event that doses are increased to a level where the patient becomes sedated but still complains of pain, it should be explained that further opioid cannot safely be given. In some patients the pain may not be completely responsive to opioids, as is the case with neuropathic pain. In this case other drugs or interventional methods of pain relief may be needed (see Chapter 10).

In most cases the aim will be to discharge the patient on no more opioid than was used before admission. Sometimes it will be less.

Preferred route of opioid administration

As noted earlier, the rate of onset of effect of a drug can be influenced by its lipid solubility, dose and route of administration.

Those who abuse opioids generally seek a change in mental status and euphoria. The more rapidly this can be achieved the more desirable it becomes. In patients who exhibit aberrant drug-taking behaviors, drug and dose regimens that minimize large and rapid swings in blood levels may be preferred. For example, PCA may be preferable to larger intravenous (IV) bolus doses or intramuscular (IM) injections of an opioid.

Monitoring for effect and side effects

In general, opioid-dependent patients, especially those with chronic noncancer pain or an addiction to opioids, tend to report higher pain scores. Therefore, pain scores may not be a reliable guide to alterations in therapy and high pain scores will not always dictate further increases in opioid dose. An objective assessment of function (e.g. ability to cough, ambulate) may be a better guide to treatment in some patients.

Use of opioids in patients with a past addiction

If a patient has had an addiction to opioids in the past there may be concern that the use of opioids for analgesia will lead to the reinstatement of a craving for drugs. While local anesthetic blocks and nonsteroidal anti-inflammatory drugs (NSAIDs) may suffice in some patients, the primary concern must still be good pain relief. If opioids are indicated they should be used in effective doses because ineffective analgesia may lead to anxiety, drug-seeking behaviors and demands, as well as pain.

Naltrexone

Increasingly, patients may be prescribed naltrexone (see Chapter 2) for the treatment of addition to opioids or alcohol. It may be difficult to achieve adequate pain relief with opioid drugs, even in high doses, until the effects of naltrexone have diminished. Alternative analgesic drugs (e.g. ketamine, NSAIDs) and techniques (e.g. local anesthetic blocks) may be necessary.

Other analgesic agents and techniques

Although discussion has centered on opioid drugs, the entire range of drugs and analgesic techniques available for acute pain management may be suitable in opioid-dependent patients. In some situations where acute pain is not anticipated to be severe, local anaesthetic blocks and NSAIDs may be sufficient.

Ketamine

As noted earlier, the NMDA receptor is thought to be one of the factors involved in the development of tolerance, and NMDA receptor antagonist drugs such as ketamine may block or reverse that tolerance. For this reason, ketamine has been administered in low doses of 50–150 mg per 24 hours by IV or subcutaneous (SC) infusion in some opioid-tolerant patients, often with good effect and few, if any, side effects. Ketamine also has analgesic activity in low doses.

PREVENTION OF WITHDRAWAL SYNDROMES

If patients are unable to continue their normal chronic opioid therapy in the postoperative or post-trauma period (e.g. because they are fasting or because their 'normal' opioid is illicit), sufficient opioid must be given to cover their basal requirement in order to prevent withdrawal. Basal requirements should be provided regardless of the reported pain.

If patients have required high doses of opioid for the treatment of acute pain for more than a few days, they may also be at risk of withdrawal if the drug is abruptly stopped or doses reduced too rapidly. In general, dose reductions of about 20–25% every day or two will allow a tapering of opioid dose without signs and symptoms of withdrawal.

Clonidine

More rapid tapering can be achieved if the patient is given clonidine (an α_2-adrenergic agonist – see Chapter 7). As well as its use in the treatment of hypertension and as an analgesic agent, clonidine has been used to prevent and/or treat signs and symptoms of withdrawal. Doses may start at 50 µg three times a day (oral or SC) and can be increased as needed. However, it must be remembered that clonidine cannot be abruptly stopped because of the risk of headache, nausea, insomnia, rebound hypertension and cardiac arrhythmias.

MANAGEMENT OF WITHDRAWAL FROM OTHER DRUGS

It is not uncommon for patients who have an addiction to opioids to be addicted to other drugs (e.g. alcohol, barbiturates or benzodiazepines). Monitoring of signs and symptoms that indicate withdrawal from these drugs is suggested, and prevention or treatment regimens should be instituted as necessary.

Signs and symptoms of withdrawal from alcohol include anxiety, agitation, restlessness, sleep disturbances, nausea and vomiting, hallucinations, confusion, disorientation and convulsions. These usually occur 12–48 hours after the last intake of alcohol. Signs and symptoms of withdrawal from benzodiazepines are similar, but onset may be delayed for 1–5 days.

INVOLVEMENT OF MULTIDISCIPLINARY AND OTHER SPECIALIST TEAMS

In many of these patients, management of behavioral, psychological, medical and other factors may be needed in addition to analgesia. Assistance from other specialist teams, including chronic pain, palliative care, drug and alcohol, and psychiatric services, may be advisable.

Opioid-dependent patients may have significant emotional and psychiatric comorbidities that require treatment. Patients with cancer pain, for example, may suffer from depression. This may be exacerbated if the acute pain for which they are now being treated serves to remind them of their limited life expectancy (e.g. if pain signifies disease progression or if the operation has been for palliation only). Common comorbidities in patients who abuse drugs or alcohol are depression, anxiety and borderline personality disorders. These too can be exacerbated during the acute pain episode.

If a patient with an addiction to opioids is not already in an addiction treatment program, the immediate postoperative or post-injury period is probably not the time to discuss the various options available. It is better to gain the confidence of the patient by providing good analgesia and to leave any discussion about treatment of addiction until later.

MANAGEMENT OF PATIENTS WITH ABERRANT DRUG-TAKING BEHAVIORS

Individualized treatment plans that help with effective and safe yet compassionate treatment can benefit patients who may exhibit significant aberrant drug-taking behaviors (e.g. patients currently abusing drugs or alcohol, those who have done so in the past, and those in drug treatment programs).

These treatment plans, which should be firmly applied, may include realistic goals for analgesia (complete pain relief is usually not realistic), expected duration of treatment, plans for dose reductions and choice of drugs available. The dangers associated with tampering with equipment, or the use of illicit drugs in addition to prescribed medications, should also be explained. All medical and nursing staff involved in treating the patient should agree to the plans. It should also be discussed with the patient.

SPECIFIC ANALGESIC TECHNIQUES

PATIENT-CONTROLLED ANALGESIA

Addiction to opioids was initially believed to be a contraindication to the use of PCA. However, it is now recognized as a potentially useful method of providing pain relief in these patients. This is partly because of the possibility of large opioid requirements and partly because it helps avoid confrontations between staff and patients about pain relief.

The central assumptions behind the use of PCA are that a patient will self-administer opioid when uncomfortable and when comfort is achieved will make no further demands. The advantages of PCA are lost if the patient uses the pump simply to self-administer as much opioid as the settings allow. The patient should be reminded to use PCA for pain control only and not for other reasons.

PCA parameters

If patients are unable to continue their normal chronic opioid medication (e.g. because they are fasting), a continuous (background) infusion can be used to cover this basal requirement, allowing for incomplete cross-tolerance where appropriate.

Larger-than-average bolus doses will often be needed, although it can be difficult to know the optimal starting dose. In some centers the size of the usual bolus dose (that is, the dose used for opioid-naive patients) is increased by 50–100%. Another method is to base the size of the bolus dose (as well as any background infusion) on the patient's normal (preadmission) opioid requirement. Examples of this are given below.

Examples of PCA orders

These examples are based on patients in whom good pain relief was obtained when 'standard' PCA protocols were adapted to suit that patient. The dose regimens are suggestions only. They may not be suitable for all patients or in all situations. The use of higher bolus doses is best limited to situations where the patient is being managed by specialist pain services, when there is 24-hour (appropriate) medical cover, when nursing and medical staff have had appropriate education and experience, and when adequate monitoring of the patient is available.

Example I

Following laparotomy, a patient is offered morphine PCA. For the last 8 months he has been taking 300 mg of a controlled-release oral morphine preparation (in divided doses) daily. He is not permitted any oral intake after the operation.

basal opioid requirement	= 300 mg/day oral morphine
using a 3:1 conversion	= 100 mg/day IV morphine
	= 4 mg/h approximately
therefore, appropriate	
background infusion	= 4 mg/h
appropriate bolus dose	= 4 mg

Doses and infusion rates may require adjustment (up or down) according to pain relief or side effects. As a general rule it may be best to keep the rate of infusion (in mg/h) the same as or less than the size of the bolus dose (in mg), so that PCA remains predominantly 'patient-controlled'.

Once the patient is tolerating unlimited oral fluids, his usual controlled-release morphine can be restarted to replace the background infusion. In addition, short-term use of immediate-release opioids, such as morphine syrup, oxycodone or hydromorphone may be needed until his total opioid requirements have decreased to a level where he can manage on his controlled-release morphine only. High PCA dose requirements may mean that there is a delay before the patient can be managed with oral opioids alone.

Example 2

A patient will receive morphine PCA after surgery for multiple injuries. For the last 6 months he has been taking 800 mg of a controlled-release oral morphine preparation (in divided doses) daily. He is not permitted any oral intake after the operation.

basal opioid requirement	=	800 mg/day oral morphine
	=	260 mg/day IV morphine approximately
	=	10 mg/h approximately

It is thought appropriate to use another opioid in the immediate postoperative period (see previous comments about incomplete cross-tolerance and morphine metabolites). The decision is made to use fentanyl.

The equianalgesic dose of 10 mg morphine would normally be considered to be about 150–200 µg fentanyl (see Chapter 2), but as cross-tolerance is likely to be incomplete doses of 50% of the equianalgesic dose are used initially, therefore:

appropriate background infusion	= 100 µg/h approximately
appropriate bolus dose	= 100 µg

Example 3

A patient is provided with morphine PCA after spinal surgery. He is not permitted any oral intake after the operation. He admits to injecting about $100 worth of heroin a day (he says this buys about 250 mg of impure heroin). He is convinced, because of his addiction and from past experience, that no one will take his pain complaints seriously and that he will have severe pain for days.

The hospital drug rehabilitation service says that the current purity of heroin in the streets is about 50–60%. The decision is made to use PCA morphine using doses appropriate to the patient's daily intake of heroin.

basal opioid requirement	=	250 mg/day impure IV heroin
if purity is about 50%	=	120 mg/day pure IV heroin
	=	240 mg/day IV morphine
	=	10 mg/h morphine (approximate values)

As the purity of the heroin cannot be verified it is decided to commence on a more conservative dose. The PCA machine is programmed to deliver a background infusion of 6 mg/h and a bolus dose of 6 mg. The patient obtains good pain relief (without side effects) using nearly 650 mg morphine in the first 24 hours after surgery. Plans for duration of treatment and progressive dose reductions are discussed.

REGIONAL ANALGESIA

A variety of regional analgesic techniques, including epidural and intrathecal analgesia, and continuous brachial plexus or lumbar plexus blocks, may be used to provide safe and effective pain relief in opioid-dependent patients.

Replacement of basal opioid requirements will be needed in order to prevent signs and symptoms of opioid withdrawal. If an opioid is added to the epidural infusion, the amount delivered may or may not be adequate for this purpose and this should be calculated for every patient. The amount of opioid administered for intrathecal analgesia (commonly 0.1–0.2 mg morphine) will be inadequate.

REFERENCES AND FURTHER READING

Collett B.J. (1998) Opioid tolerance: the clinical perspective. *British Journal of Anaesthesia* **81**, 58–68.

Lawlor P.G. and Bruera E. (1998) Side effects of opioids in chronic pain treatment. *Current Opinion in Anaesthesiology* **11**, 539–545.

Mercadante S. (1999) Opioid rotation for cancer pain: rationale and clinical aspects. *Cancer* **86**, 1856–1865.

National Health and Medical Research Council (1999) *Acute Pain Management: The Scientific Evidence.* Canberra (available at http://www.nhmrc.health.gov.au/publicat/pdf/cp57.pdf).

O'Brien C.P. (1996) Drug addiction and drug abuse. In *Goodman and Gilman's The Pharmacological Basis of Therapeutics*, 9th edition (eds Hardman G.H., Goodman Gilman A. and Limbird L.E). McGraw-Hill, New York.

Passik S.D. and Portenoy R.K. (1998) Substance abuse issues. In *The Management of Pain* (eds Ashburn M.A. and Rice L.J.). Churchill Livingstone, Philadelphia.

Porter J. and Jick H. (1980) Addiction rare in patients treated with narcotics. *New England Journal of Medicine* **302**, 123.

Rapp S.E., Ready L.B. and Nessly M.L. (1995) Acute pain management in patients with prior opioid consumption: a case-controlled retrospective review. *Pain* **61**, 195–201.

Ready L.B. and Laird D. (1998) The interface between acute and chronic pain. In *The Management of Pain* (eds Ashburn M.A. and Rice L.J.). Churchill Livingstone, Philadelphia.

Silverstein J.H., Silva D.A. and Iberti T.J. (1993) Opioid addiction in anesthesiology. *Anesthesiology* **79**, 354–371.

Weisman D.E. and Haddox J.D. (1989) Opioid pseudoaddiction: an iatrogenic syndrome. *Pain* **36**, 363–366.

Zacny J.P. and Galinkin J.L. (1999) Psychotropic drugs used in anesthesia practice. *Anesthesiology* **90**, 269–288.

Chapter 10

ACUTE NEUROPATHIC PAIN

Comparison of neuropathic and nociceptive pain

Clinical features of neuropathic pain

Examples of acute neuropathic pain

Treatment of acute neuropathic pain

The role of neuropathic pain in some chronic pain states is well known. However, its role in the acute pain setting is much less well recognized. In this setting there are a small number of patients in whom neuropathic pain predominates, or contributes to the pain they are experiencing. It is often underdiagnosed and therefore undertreated.

It is important for those who look after patients with acute pain to be aware of the signs and symptoms of neuropathic pain (which might not be seen until some time after the initial injury) and to be aware of available treatment options. There will be some patients who, because of the type of surgery or nature of injury sustained, are at risk of developing neuropathic pain. Early recognition and aggressive management of these patients (possibly including pre-emptive treatment) may reduce the incidence and severity of subsequent chronic pain problems.

Provision of effective pain relief in these patients can be a difficult and challenging task and one that may be ongoing for weeks, months or even years. It is recommended that advice be obtained from specialist pain medicine physicians.

COMPARISON OF NEUROPATHIC AND NOCICEPTIVE PAIN

Pain can be broadly classified into two main types – nociceptive and neuropathic.

NOCICEPTIVE PAIN

Nociceptive pain is the most common type of pain seen in acute clinical care and its treatment is therefore the primary focus of this book. It results from stimulation of specialized sensory nerve endings (called nociceptors) as a consequence of tissue damage or inflammation (e.g. after surgery, infection or trauma). Central sensitization involving the N-methyl-D-aspartate (NMDA) receptor (see Chapter 7) may develop.

NEUROPATHIC PAIN

Neuropathic pain is pain associated with injury or disease of the peripheral or central nervous system. Following such injury, a number of changes occur at the peripheral and/or spinal cord levels, including the development of central sensitization, reorganization of synaptic connections in the spinal cord, and hyperexcitability of damaged peripheral nerves. As a result of these changes the patient may exhibit signs and symptoms which are typical of neuropathic pain (**Box 10.1**).

CLINICAL FEATURES OF NEUROPATHIC PAIN

The diagnosis of neuropathic pain can usually be made on the basis of a complete history and physical examination. Features that suggest neuropathic pain are listed in **Box 10.1**. They do not all have to be present in order for a diagnosis of neuropathic pain to be made.

EXAMPLES OF ACUTE NEUROPATHIC PAIN

A few of the many possible causes of neuropathic pain in the acute clinical setting are listed in **Box 10.2**.

The risk of postoperative neuropathic pain appears to be higher after some operations than others. Two commonly quoted examples are thoracotomy and mastectomy operations, where an intercostal nerve or an intercostobrachial nerve, respectively, may be damaged.

Clinical features that suggest neuropathic pain

- history of injury or disease leading to damage of peripheral nerves or spinal cord, e.g. brachial plexus avulsion, amputation of a limb, invasion of a nerve plexus by cancer, spinal cord injury, acute herpes zoster (shingles), third-degree burns
- evidence of damage to peripheral nerves or spinal cord (sensory loss, motor weakness, bowel or bladder sphincter abnormalities, reflex changes)
- evidence of increased sympathetic activity (alterations in skin color, temperature and texture, sweating, and hair and nail growth)
- a delay in the onset of pain after injury (not invariable and more likely after central injury)
- pain in an area of sensory loss (but not necessarily confined to this area)
- presence of pain that is different in nature to nociceptive pain, e.g. burning, shooting, stabbing, 'electric shocks'
- presence of pain that appears to be responding poorly to opioids
- spontaneous or paroxysmal pain
- *allodynia*: the sensation of pain in response to a stimulus that does not normally cause pain (e.g. light touch)
- *hyperalgesia*: an increased (i.e. exaggerated) response to a stimulus that is normally painful
- *dysesthesias*: unpleasant abnormal sensations
- *hyperpathia*: increasing pain with repetitive stimulation; radiation of pain to adjacent areas after stimulation; continued exacerbation of pain after stimulation ('after response')

Box 10.1
Adapted from National Health and Medical Research Council (1999).

Amputation of a limb is inevitably associated with nerve section, which can lead to a number of altered sensations. *Phantom pain* refers to painful sensations in the missing limb; *stump pain* to pain in the amputation stump; and *phantom limb* to painless sensations in the missing limb. Nerve injury (and subsequent neuropathic pain) is likely to play a major role in these ongoing pain problems. The risk of phantom pain appears

Examples of neuropathic pain in the acute pain setting

Postoperative
- post-thoracotomy
- post-mastectomy
- post-amputation

Post-trauma
- spinal cord injury
- post-amputation
- third-degree burns
- brachial plexus avulsion
- sacral root injury in association with a fractured pelvis
- major crush injuries of upper or lower limbs

Associated with cancer
- pancreatic cancer (involvement of the celiac plexus)
- compression of the brachial plexus after spread of lung cancer to apical lymph nodes
- involvement of sacral nerve roots by pelvic lymph node metastases

Associated with medical illnesses
- viral infections, e.g. acute herpes zoster (shingles)/post-herpetic neuralgia, HIV/AIDS
- diabetic neuropathy
- alcoholic neuropathy
- demyelinating diseases such as multiple sclerosis

Box 10.2

to be increased if severe pain existed prior to amputation, whereas cause (elective or traumatic), level of amputation, age and gender appear not to influence the risk.

Neuropathic pain may also occur after burn injuries. The belief that third-degree burns are not painful is inaccurate; damaged nerve endings may result in neuropathic pain in the post-acute phase.

COMPLEX REGIONAL PAIN SYNDROME

Complex regional pain syndrome (CRPS) is another form of neuropathic pain that is associated with abnormalities of the sympathetic nervous system. The clinical features of CRPS include changes in motor function; spontaneous and/or burning pain, allodynia and hyperalgesia; atrophy of skin, hair and nails; and autonomic changes (alteration in skin blood flow, edema and excessive sweating).

Type 1 CRPS (previously referred to as 'reflex sympathetic dystrophy') results in the features listed above and a neuropathic-like pain that exists in the absence of detectable nerve injury. The term CRPS type 2 (previously referred to as 'causalgia') is used when these features occur after nerve injury.

TREATMENT OF ACUTE NEUROPATHIC PAIN

Treatment of neuropathic pain may require a combination of pharmacologic, physical and behavioral therapy. However, in the acute stage, it usually begins with drug therapy (**Box 10.3**) and/or the use of regional neural blockade. Effective analgesia is often difficult to achieve and may require the use of a number of different drugs or techniques. These are often added in a stepwise manner as needed at intervals of a few days, so that the effectiveness of each addition can be seen.

It is known that for some patients, early recognition and aggressive management of acute neuropathic pain may reduce the risk or severity of subsequent chronic neuropathic pain. Possible treatment regimens include regional neural blockade (e.g. continuous epidural or brachial plexus analgesia) and the use of NMDA receptor antagonists (e.g. ketamine), tricyclic antidepressants, anticonvulsants and antiarrhythmics. A combination of these therapies may be more effective than one therapy alone.

PRE-EMPTIVE TREATMENT

Pre-emptive treatment, aimed at preventing the onset of central sensitization, may also be effective. For example, the use of

Pharmacological options for the treatment of acute neuropathic pain

Drugs	Examples
Opioids*	Methadone, morphine, oxycodone, tramadol
Tricyclic antidepressants	Amitriptyline, nortriptyline, imipramine, dothiepin, doxepin
NMDA receptor antagonists	Ketamine
Anticonvulsants	Carbamazepine, sodium valproate, phenytoin, gabapentin
Antiarrhythmics	Lidocaine (lignocaine), mexiletine
Alpha-2-adrenergic agonists	Clonidine
Topical agents	Capsaicin, lidocaine

Box 10.3

*Neuropathic pain is typically less responsive to opioids than nociceptive pain.

epidural analgesia to relieve preoperative limb pain and provide effective postoperative pain relief has been shown to reduce the risk of phantom pain after lower limb amputation. It has also been shown that if patients with acute herpes zoster are treated with amitriptyline at an early stage in the disease, the risk of postherpetic neuralgia (a severe form of neuropathic pain) can be significantly reduced.

In patients thought to be at risk of neuropathic pain after surgery or injury, it may be worth initiating therapy *before* any clinical features of neuropathic pain develop. For example, if a young patient is admitted following traumatic amputation of an arm, pre-emptive treatment could be considered. An example of a pre-emptive regimen that might be used for such a patient is amitriptyline 25 mg at night, an intravenous (IV) ketamine infusion at 100–150 mg/day (for 5–7 days), and morphine by patient-controlled analgesia (PCA) or a continuous brachial plexus block using a local anesthetic infusion (for 4–6 days). Even if neuropathic pain does not develop while the patient is in hospital, it may be worth continuing the amitriptyline for 3 months.

OPIOIDS

Neuropathic pain is often regarded as unresponsive to opioids, but this may not be so in all cases. It is however, typically less responsive than nociceptive pain. One of the early signs of development of neuropathic pain in the acute situation is a lack of apparent pain relief despite increasing doses of opioid, and possibly the onset of sedation in a patient who still reports high pain scores.

TRICYCLIC ANTIDEPRESSANTS

Tricyclic antidepressants (TCAs) are commonly used as first-line agents in the treatment of neuropathic pain and have been shown to be effective in a variety of neuropathic pain states. The analgesic effect of these drugs is believed to be distinct from the effect on mood, as pain relief can be obtained in the absence of depression. These drugs may also help 'normalize' sleep patterns. Effects on pain and sleep are likely to be seen at relatively low doses and within a few days of starting treatment, whereas antidepressant effects may require several weeks and higher doses.

Mechanism of action

Tricyclic antidepressants inhibit reuptake of monoamines into nerve terminals and modulate pain sensation via descending inhibitory pathways in the spinal cord. Older generation TCAs (e.g. amitriptyline, imipramine), which inhibit reuptake of norepinephrine (noradrenaline) and serotonin (5-hydroxy-tryptamine, 5HT), appear to be the most effective in the treatment of neuropathic pain. Newer serotonin-selective reuptake inhibitors (SSRIs), which inhibit reuptake of serotonin only, may have fewer side effects but have not been shown to be as effective. The TCAs also block sodium channels and α_2-adrenergic receptors, and these actions may contribute to their analgesic effects.

Amitriptyline is probably the most widely used and studied TCA of those used in chronic pain states. Its major metabolite, nortriptyline, has analgesic activity. Amitriptyline has also been shown to have NMDA receptor antagonist properties.

Side effects

Side effects of TCAs result mainly from their anticholinergic actions. They include dry mouth, increased heart rate, blurred vision, constipation and urinary retention. Narrow-angle glaucoma may be aggravated and arrhythmias can occur. Impairment of cardiac conduction has been reported (usually of ore importance in overdose). These drugs may be contraindicated in patients with pre-existing cardiac conduction abnormalities. Sedation is reasonably common.

Elderly patients may be more at risk of postural (orthostatic) hypotension, dysphoria, agitation and confusion. Other more serious side effects are rare but include bone marrow depression, skin rashes and hepatic dysfunction.

Clinical use

Since tolerance develops to both the anticholinergic and sedative effects of TCAs, it is common to start TCAs at a low, single daily dose and to increase the dose every few days as required. As TCAs may cause drowsiness, especially in the early stages of treatment, doses are best given at night.

Commonly used starting doses for amitriptyline are 10 mg in patients over 60 years old and 25 mg in those younger than 60 years. Doses may be increased by 10 mg or 25 mg (depending on patient age) every 3–5 days if required. A satisfactory response usually occurs at levels between 25 mg and 100 mg, although higher doses may sometimes be needed. Alternative TCAs include dothiepin, doxepin, imipramine and desimipramine.

Care must be taken if the patient is already taking an SSRI. If TCAs are also needed, doses should be reduced and the patient monitored closely for any side effects.

NMDA RECEPTOR ANTAGONISTS

There is evidence for NMDA receptor involvement in central sensitization and neuropathic pain. An IV infusion of ketamine, an NMDA receptor antagonist (see Chapter 7), may give immediate relief in some forms of this pain.

ANTICONVULSANTS

Anticonvulsant drugs have been shown to be effective in a variety of neuropathic pain states. They are thought to work by blocking sodium channels and stabilizing cell membranes ('membrane stabilizers'), thus reducing spontaneous and evoked neuronal activity. They are often used when TCAs alone have failed to produce adequate analgesia.

Carbamazepine

Carbamazepine is structurally related to imipramine. It is often commenced at low doses (e.g. 50–100 mg orally 12-hourly) and increased after a few days if required and if there are no side effects. The range of doses needed to treat neuropathic pain is unknown, but the effective dose is often less than that necessary for seizure control.

Side effects are reasonably common. During long-term treatment, the most frequently reported side effects are blurred vision, drowsiness, ataxia and vertigo. Other possible adverse effects include nausea and vomiting, blood dyscrasias, hepatic dysfunction and rashes.

Sodium valproate

Sodium valproate is another anticonvulsant that may be useful in the treatment of neuropathic pain. Side effects are probably less common than with carbamazepine but include nausea, rashes, ataxia, hepatic dysfunction and thrombocytopenia.

Gabapentin

Gabapentin is a newer anticonvulsant drug that does not cause blood dyscrasias. Its mechanism of action remains unclear.

ANTIARRHYTHMICS

Antiarrhythmic drugs are also thought to work by blocking sodium channels and stabilizing cell membranes.

Lidocaine (lignocaine)

A single dose of IV lidocaine (1–5 mg/kg over 30–120 minutes) can be given to test the effectiveness of this drug. If successful it may be followed by an IV or subcutaneous infusion (0.5–1.5 mg/kg per hour) or a trial of mexiletine. Analgesia from a single dose may exceed by days or weeks the known pharmacological duration of action of the drug. The mechanism of action is unclear but it does not appear to involve blockade of peripheral nerves. Ectopic impulses generated by damaged nerves appear to be blocked at concentrations of local anesthetic that are lower than those normally required to block nerve impulses.

Mexiletine

Mexiletine is an antiarrhythmic drug that is structurally related to lidocaine but can be given orally. Side effects include nausea, sedation and tremor. Care should be taken in patients with ischemic heart disease or cardiac arrhythmias.

ALPHA-2-ADRENERGIC AGONISTS

Clonidine, an α_2 agonist (see Chapter 7) has also been used in the management of neuropathic pain.

TOPICAL AGENTS

Topical agents may be useful when allodynia is a prominent component of neuropathic pain. The most widely used for this purpose is *capsaicin* (the active ingredient of hot chilli peppers). It is available as a cream that is applied to the painful area several times a day. Its analgesic effect is believed to result from the depletion of substance P (a neurotransmitter) in unmyelinated sensory nerves, which then leads to a block of these nerves. When applied to the skin, capsaicin first induces a burning feeling and hyperalgesia.

There may also be possible benefits from the application of topical anesthetic agents including lidocaine (see Chapter 3). Topical applications of aspirin or other NSAIDs in chloroform or ether suspension have also been reported to be of some benefit.

REGIONAL NEURAL BLOCKADE

A variety of regional and sympathetic blocks may be of use in the treatment of neuropathic pain. For example, epidural analgesia may prevent or reduce neuropathic pain following lower limb amputation; a celiac plexus block might be useful in the treatment of pain due to pancreatic cancer; a stellate ganglion block may help in the management of CRPS of the arm; and continuous brachial plexus blockade may be used following upper limb amputation.

TRANSCUTANEOUS ELECTRICAL NERVE STIMULATION

Transcutaneous electrical nerve stimulation (see Chapter 8) can also be useful, especially if stimulation of the nerve trunk is possible proximal to the site of injury.

REFERENCES AND FURTHER READING

Bach S., Noreng M.F. and Tjellden N.U. (1988) Phantom limb in amputees during the first 12 months following limb amputation after preoperative lumbar epidural blockade. *Pain* **33**, 297–310.

Bryson H.M. and Wilde M.I. (1996) Amitriptyline: a review of its pharmacological properties and therapeutic use in chronic pain states. *Drugs and Aging* **8**, 459–476.

Dellemijn P. (1999) Are opioids effective in relieving neuropathic pain? *Pain* **80**, 453–462.

Fields H.L., Baron R. and Rowbotham M.C. (1999) Peripheral neuropathic pain: an approach to management. In *The Textbook of Pain* (eds Wall P.D. and Melzack R.). Churchill Livingstone, Edinburgh.

Hayes C. and Molloy A.R. (1997) Neuropathic pain in the postoperative period. *International Anesthesiology Clinics* **35**, 67–91.

Karlsten R. and Gordh T. (1997) How do drugs relieve neurogenic pain? *Drugs and Aging* **11**, 398–412.

National Health and Medical Research Council (1999) *Acute Pain Management: The Scientific Evidence*. Canberra (available at http://www.nhmrc.health.gov.au/publicat/pdf/cp57.pdf).

Sindrup S.H. and Jensen T.S. (1999) Efficacy of pharmacological treatments of neuropathic pain: an update and effect related to mechanism of drug action. *Pain* **82**, 389–400.

Tryba M. (1998) Prevention of chronic pain syndromes by anaesthetic measures: fact or fiction? *Baillière's Clinical Anaesthesiology* **12**, 133–143.

Woolf C.J. (1995) Somatic pain – pathogenesis and prevention. *British Journal of Anaesthesia* **75**, 169–176.

CHAPTER 11

THE ELDERLY PATIENT

Changes in pharmacokinetics and pharmacodynamics

Assessment of pain

Analgesic drugs

Analgesic techniques

Advances in anesthesia and surgery, combined with the increasing proportion of elderly people in the populations of most countries, mean that greater numbers of older patients are now presenting for major operations. These patients are at higher risk of complications from surgery and from unrelieved or undertreated acute pain (see Chapter 1). They are therefore particularly likely to benefit from effective pain relief. However, a number of a factors may combine to make control of pain more difficult than in the younger patient. These include:

- age-related alterations in pharmacokinetics (how the individual deals with the drug) and pharmacodynamics (how the individual responds to the drug)
- diminished physiological reserves
- concurrent diseases
- altered pain responses and difficulties in the assessment of pain
- concurrent medications, leading to an increased risk of drug interactions

CHANGES IN PHARMACOKINETICS AND PHARMACODYNAMICS

PHARMACOKINETICS

The pharmacokinetics (absorption, distribution, metabolism and excretion) of many drugs are altered in the elderly. This is due primarily to two factors – the progressive physiological decline that occurs with increasing age and the increasing likelihood of concurrent disease.

Age-related physiological changes

The physiological changes associated with aging are progressive, but the rate of decline can be highly variable between individuals (i.e. physiological aging may or may not parallel chronological aging). It is also difficult to separate changes due to age and those that result from the higher incidence of degenerative and other diseases that is inevitable in this age group. The physiological changes associated with aging that are of most significance to pharmacokinetics are those related to cardiac output, liver and renal function, and protein binding.

Cardiac output

Cardiac output is an important determinant of the blood concentration of a drug, particularly after administration of an intravenous (IV) bolus dose. Cardiac output may decrease by up to 20% as a result of aging. As a consequence, peak blood concentrations reached after a single IV bolus in an elderly patient are likely to be higher than in a younger patient given the same dose. To compensate, the dose of drug should be decreased and/or the dose given more slowly.

Hepatic function

Liver size and hepatic blood flow are decreased by as much as 25–40% in the elderly. For drugs that depend on the liver for metabolism (e.g. most opioids), a 25–40% reduction in clearance may therefore be expected. Unlike the changes in cardiac output, this will have little effect on blood concentrations following a single IV bolus dose, but may lead to higher steady state blood levels if drugs are administered repeatedly or continuously (e.g. by infusion). This means that the maintenance doses of drugs that are dependent on the liver for clearance may need to be decreased.

The activity of some liver enzymes may also be reduced by up to 25%. Those responsible for demethylation decline rapidly with aging, which in turn may slow the clearance of drugs such as diazepam.

Renal function

The greatest physiological change associated with aging is reduction in renal function. Renal blood flow may decrease by more than 10% per decade and glomerular filtration rate and creatinine clearance may be reduced by 30–50% and 50–70% respectively in the older patient. For these reasons, it has been suggested that elderly patients should be considered to be renally impaired, even if blood urea and creatinine levels remain within 'normal' laboratory ranges.

Diminished renal function reduces the clearance of drugs or drug metabolites (e.g. the metabolites of morphine and normeperidine) which rely on the kidney for excretion, leading to an increase in steady state blood concentrations. Maintenance doses of such drugs may therefore need to be decreased, or drugs that have active metabolites avoided.

Increasing body fat, decreasing muscle mass

Aging is associated with an increase in body fat at the expense of reduced muscle mass. However, this may not result in clinically significant changes in pharmacokinetics.

Altered protein binding

There is an age-related change in plasma protein levels. This may alter plasma concentration of the free ('active') fraction of a drug and therefore the dose requirements of some drugs. For example, the reduced dose requirement for diazepam in the elderly is associated with age-related decreases in albumin concentration.

Absorption

Absorption of drugs from oral, intramuscular (IM) and subcutaneous (SC) routes is relatively unchanged in the elderly.

Concurrent diseases

A wide variety of degenerative and other diseases (which have an increasing prevalence in the elderly) and concurrent use of other drugs may alter the factors outlined above. For example, congestive cardiac failure and chronic liver disease may be associated with reductions in hepatic blood flow.

PHARMACODYNAMICS

Age-related changes in pharmacodynamics also occur, although the mechanisms behind these changes are poorly understood. It appears that the sensitivity of the brain to opioids is increased by about 50% in the elderly. However, it is not clear whether this difference is due to alterations in the number and/or function of opioid receptors in the central nervous system, or whether it is due to other factors.

ASSESSMENT OF PAIN

It is commonly believed that elderly patients perceive less pain than younger patients. Elderly patients may report no pain, or less pain, in conditions that are usually associated with severe pain such as myocardial infarction and intra-abdominal emergencies. The significance of these events (i.e. whether or not they truly represent changes in pain perception) and the mechanisms behind them are unclear. Studies using experimental pain have shown mixed results. It is possible that significant age-related changes in pain perception do not occur.

When pain is reported, it should receive as much attention in the elderly (regardless of any possible changes in pain perception) as in the younger patient. Even though older patients may not voluntarily report pain, pain should be presumed to exist if the situation is potentially painful.

The assessment of pain and evaluation of pain relief therapies may be more difficult in the elderly patient owing to differences in reporting of pain, cognitive impairment, and difficulties in measurement.

REPORTING OF PAIN

Many factors may lead to under-reporting of pain in elderly patients. These include psychological and cultural factors such as fear, anxiety, depression, cognitive impairment, the implication of the disease, loss of independence, feelings of isolation, the quality of social support available, and family. The elderly and their carers may even see pain as a normal part of aging.

COGNITIVE IMPAIRMENT

Cognitive function declines with age and patients who have cognitive impairment are known to be at greater risk of undertreatment of acute pain. This may be due, in part, to under-reporting. The reasons for this are not clear but it could result from factors such as memory impairment, diminished pain perception, or diminished capacity to report pain. There is also a tendency among staff and carers to disbelieve the pain complaints of confused or delirious patients.

Delirium (or confusion) is a common form of acute cognitive impairment. In the elderly patient it is reasonably common during acute illnesses or in the postoperative period. While the exact cause may be unknown, a number of risk factors have been identified (**Box 11.1**). If a patient becomes confused while taking opioids, a common reaction is to stop the opioid. However, as

Risk factors for the development of delirium

- old age
- pre-existing dementia
- anticholinergic drugs (including some antiemetics), psychoactive drugs, benzodiazepines, opioids
- withdrawal from alcohol or sedatives
- infection
- fluid and electrolyte imbalance
- hypoxemia
- severe pain
- multiple concurrent medical problems
- multiple concurrent medications

Box 11.1

confusion may be the result of many other factors, consideration should be given to simply reducing the dose of opioid rather than complete avoidance of the drug.

MEASUREMENT OF PAIN

Accurate and repeated assessments of pain are necessary for effective pain management. As with younger patients, the elderly patient's self-report is the most reliable indicator of pain.

Measures of pain in common use in the acute pain setting, such as the visual analog scale (VAS), verbal numerical rating scale (VNRS) and verbal descriptor scale (VDS) (see Chapter 1) have all been used for assessment of pain in the elderly. Compared with VAS and VNRS, the VDS (which uses familiar words such as 'none', 'slight', 'mild', 'moderate', 'severe' and 'extreme') may be more reliable.

Patients with mild to moderate cognitive impairment may need to be given more time to think about and respond to questions, and repeated questioning may be required. These patients are often able to assess pain reliably at the time when asked (present pain), but recall of pain (e.g. if asked about pain over the last few days or weeks) may be less reliable.

In noncommunicative patients assessment of pain can be more difficult. Commonly, behaviors such as restlessness, tense muscles, frowning or grimacing, and grunting or groaning, are used to assess pain severity. However, there may be other reasons for such behavior.

Observation of function, such as the ability to take deep breaths and cough, as well as tolerate physiotherapy and walking, is also important and may help to assess adequacy of analgesia.

ANALGESIC DRUGS

As with younger patients, a range of analgesic drugs may be used in the management of acute nociceptive and neuropathic pain. These drugs are covered in more detail in previous chapters. The comments that follow relate primarily to differences in their use or effects in the elderly.

In general, adverse effects of drugs are more common in the elderly. They include drug–drug, disease–drug and adverse drug reactions.

OPIOIDS

If opioids are to be used effectively yet safely in the elderly patient, a number of factors must be considered (**Box 11.2**).

Suitable opioid drugs and preparations

Pure opioid agonists are usually the drugs of choice in the elderly patient. Drugs with a short half-life (e.g. morphine) are preferred as this facilitates rapid titration of dose. Agonist-antagonist opioids (e.g. butorphanol and nalbuphine) are generally not recommended because of a higher incidence of delirium.

Choice of opioid preparation is also important. Rapid titration is not possible using preparations designed to allow a slow and sustained release of opioid, such as sustained-release oral morphine preparations and transdermal fentanyl patches. In addition, the persistent drug levels and slow offset of these preparations can make any side effects difficult to treat. They are not generally recommended for acute pain management and may be particularly problematic in the elderly opioid-naive patient.

Considerations for safe and effective use of opioids in the elderly patient

- use of a suitable opioid
- use of a suitable opioid preparation
- awareness of potential problems with opioid metabolites
- age-related dose schedules
- adequate monitoring and careful titration to effect
- avoidance of concurrent use of sedatives
- recognition and appropriate treatment of opioid-related side effects

Box 11.2

Opioid metabolites

Accumulation of morphine 6-glucuronide (M6G) and morphine 3-glucuronide (M3G) may occur as a result of impaired renal function and decreased renal clearance. The increase in M6G levels may necessitate unexpectedly low maintenance doses of morphine, owing to the analgesic activity of M6G. Unless large doses of morphine are required, problems due to accumulation of M3G (see Chapter 2) are unlikely to be seen in the acute pain setting. Meperidine (pethidine) is probably best avoided in the elderly because significant accumulation of the active metabolite, normeperidine, may occur. Accumulation of the metabolites of propoxyphene may lead to confusion, delusions and hallucinations in the older patient. In patients with renal impairment, a drug without active metabolites, such as fentanyl, may be a useful alternative.

Opioid dose and dose intervals

Opioid requirements decrease with increasing patient age. The reasons for this have not been fully explained, as noted in Chapter 2. Although total daily opioid doses are likely to be less than those needed by younger patients, elderly patients will still exhibit the wide interpatient variability in opioid dose and in blood levels required for effective analgesia.

Fixed-interval dosing may not allow the flexibility required to individualize treatment. However, although PRN schedules can provide this flexibility, it should not be left to the elderly patient to request analgesia. Pain must be assessed, and analgesia offered, on a regular basis.

While effective duration of a single dose may be increased in the elderly, in the absence of any contraindication, these patients should not be denied further doses solely because duration of action is expected to be prolonged.

Titration of opioids

Titration is discussed in detail in Chapter 2 and the same principles apply to the elderly patient.

Side effects of opioids

Respiratory depression

The fear of causing respiratory depression in the elderly patient often leads to inadequate doses of opioid being given. As with other patients, significant respiratory depression can generally be avoided if appropriate monitoring is in place.

Hypoxemia

The elderly are at particular risk of hypoxemia in the postoperative period. There are a number of contributing factors including pre-existing disease, the surgery itself, and the respiratory effects of opioids (see Chapter 2). The elderly patient is also likely to be at higher risk from the possible adverse effects of hypoxemia, such as myocardial ischemia and infarction, cognitive impairment and confusion. Supplemental oxygen may minimize the risk of significant hypoxemia and it is sometimes recommended for the first 48–72 hours following major surgery, regardless of the method of opioid administration.

Nausea and vomiting

The incidence of nausea and vomiting in the postoperative period decreases with increasing age. Routine administration of antiemetics is not recommended, as some of these drugs (particularly those with anticholinergic properties) are more likely to cause side effects in the elderly.

Pruritus

Pruritus appears to be less common in the elderly.

Cognitive effects

Compared with morphine, fentanyl may cause less postoperative confusion and less change in cognitive function.

Tramadol

The elimination half-life of tramadol is known to be slightly prolonged in elderly patients and therefore lower daily doses may be required. However, there remains a paucity of clinical data regarding the use of this drug in elderly patients.

LOCAL ANESTHETIC DRUGS

Clearance of local anesthetic drugs may be decreased in elderly patients. If repeat doses or continuous infusions are used, the total dose should be reduced in order to avoid possible accumulation. Infusions of local anesthetic solution in combination with low concentrations of an opioid such as fentanyl may enable the amount of local anesthetic drug to be reduced.

NONSTEROIDAL ANTI-INFLAMMATORY DRUGS

Elderly patients are more likely to have renal impairment, cardiac failure and hypovolemia, or to be using diuretic or anti-hypertensive medications. This puts them at increased risk of renal complications due to administration of nonsteroidal anti-inflammatory drugs (NSAIDs). They are also more at risk of gastrointestinal side effects. The incidence of side effects is increased when NSAIDs with longer half-lives are used, so these are probably best avoided in the elderly patient. In frail elderly patients NSAIDs may cause cognitive impairment.

Newer NSAIDs that selectively inhibit COX-2 produce fewer side effects and may be a better choice in the elderly patient.

Acetaminophen (paracetamol)

There is no consistent evidence regarding the effect of aging on clearance of acetaminophen and there may be no need to reduce doses in the elderly.

ADJUVANT ANALGESIC DRUGS

Tricyclic antidepressants

Elderly patients are particularly prone to the side effects of tricyclic antidepressants (TCAs), such as sedation, confusion, orthostatic hypotension, dry mouth, constipation and urinary retention. They are also more likely to have diseases that require TCAs to be administered with caution (e.g. prostatic hypertrophy, narrow-angle glaucoma, cardiovascular disease and impaired liver function).

Clearance of TCAs may be reduced in the elderly patient. Low doses should be prescribed initially with gradual increases if required.

Anticonvulsants

Elderly patients are more likely to develop side effects from anticonvulsant drugs. Initial doses should be lower than for younger patients and any increases should be titrated slowly. Age-related reductions in liver function may affect elimination of drugs such as carbamazepine. Age-related decreases in renal function may affect the clearance of drugs dependent on the kidney for excretion (e.g. gabapentin).

ANALGESIC TECHNIQUES

The management of some analgesic techniques may need to be adapted for elderly patients. These techniques are covered in detail in previous chapters and the comments that follow relate primarily to the differences in their use or effects in the elderly.

INTERMITTENT OPIOID ADMINISTRATION

Intermittent injections and oral administration of opioids continue to be the mainstays of treatment in elderly patients in the acute pain setting. As in younger patients, their effectiveness can be improved if suitable titration regimens are used. Details of these regimens are outlined in Chapter 4 and are applicable to patients of all ages. It must be stressed that PRN regimens, while they may allow greater flexibility, should not rely on the elderly patient requesting medication. Instead, staff should offer pain relief at frequent intervals.

CONTINUOUS IV OR SC INFUSIONS

Continuous infusions are often used in an attempt to avoid the peaks and troughs in blood concentration associated with intermittent administration. However, it is difficult to predict the required blood level for any particular patient. Since elderly patients may have low opioid requirements and as there may be difficulties in assessment of pain, degree of pain relief, and opioid-related side effects, continuous infusions are probably the least safe way of giving opioids to the elderly patient.

PATIENT-CONTROLLED ANALGESIA

Patient-controlled analgesia (PCA) should not be withheld from elderly patients simply because of their age. As long as there are no contraindications to the use of PCA (see Chapter 5) and as long as the patient is able to comprehend the technique, PCA may be a safe and effective form of pain relief. Although in general the proportion of elderly patients who can effectively use PCA will be less than in younger age groups, some patients in their nineties have been reported to use PCA successfully. Elderly patients should be followed closely to ensure that they understand the concept of self-administration and to ensure that they are obtaining adequate pain relief.

In the elderly patient (over 70 years) it is suggested that the size of the PCA bolus dose be reduced. If pain relief is inadequate the number of bolus doses that have been delivered should be checked. If the patient is making few successful demands an increase in the size of the bolus dose may be inappropriate. The patient will either need further education or an alternative form of analgesia. If the patient is making many successful demands an increase in the size of the bolus dose may be required.

The use of a background infusion (continuous infusion) with PCA has been shown to increase the amount of opioid delivered and increase the risk of side effects. Therefore, their use in elderly patients should be avoided. The opioid-tolerant patient may be an exception.

It is wise to avoid concurrent use of drugs that depress the central nervous system, especially longer-acting sedatives such as scopolamine (hyoscine) and lorazepam. As well as the risk of respiratory depression in any patient receiving opioids, they can reduce the chance of older patients remembering what they have been told about PCA and therefore their ability to understand and use PCA appropriately. This therapy should be stopped if a patient becomes confused, as it may no longer be used correctly.

EPIDURAL ANALGESIA

Elderly patients are at particular risk of complications after surgery or major trauma and they are therefore most likely to benefit from an analgesic technique, such as epidural analgesia, that can improve outcome (see Chapter 6). If closely supervised by an acute pain service team, with appropriate patient monitoring and staff education, even elderly patients (including those over 100 years old) with epidural analgesia can be safely managed in general surgical wards.

As with parenteral opioids, epidural opioid requirements decrease with increasing patient age. In addition, the spread of local anesthetic drug in the epidural space is greater in the elderly, meaning that smaller volumes of local anesthetic solution will be needed. Whether these drugs are used alone or in combination, age-based dose or infusion rate regimens should be used.

The elderly may be more at risk of some of the adverse effects of epidural analgesia (e.g. they may be less able to compensate for hypovolemia). They may also be less likely to mention side effects such as motor or sensory block or backache, which could indicate an epidural hematoma or abscess. Therefore, they need close monitoring. As with any patient, minimization of hemodynamic change (including orthostatic hypotension), early ambulation, and early recognition of any major complication will be made easier if analgesia is titrated to provide sufficient pain relief without motor and sensory block. Appropriate placement of the epidural catheter will help to reduce the dose of drugs required for effective pain relief, and therefore help to minimize side effects.

It should be noted that dose and duration of effect of anticoagulant drugs can be altered in the elderly. This may be clinically important when these drugs are used in patients receiving epidural analgesia. In the elderly patient, low molecular weight heparins are primarily eliminated by the kidney so clearance is likely to be reduced. Age-related decreases in warfarin requirements are also seen due to alterations in free plasma warfarin fractions and decreased production of clotting factors. Concurrent medical problems, including cardiac and renal disease, and interactions with other drugs (both more likely in the elderly patient) can also lead to an increased sensitivity to warfarin therapy.

REFERENCES AND FURTHER READING

Agency for Health Care Policy and Research (1992) *Acute Pain Management: Operative or Medical Procedures and Trauma. Clinical Practice Guideline.* AHCPR Pub. No. 92–0032. Rockville, MD. Agency for Health Care Policy and Research, US Department of Health and Human Services.

Bernus B., Dickinson R.G., Hooper W.D. and Eadie M.J. (1997) Anticonvulsant therapy in aged patients. Clinical pharmacokinetic considerations. *Drugs and Aging* **10**, 278–289.

Drage M.P. and Schug S.A. (1996) Analgesia in the elderly: practical treatment recommendations. *Drugs and Aging* **9**, 311–318.

Egbert A.M. (1996) Postoperative pain management in the frail elderly. *Clinics in Geriatric Medicine* **12**, 583–599.

Farrell M.J., Katz B. and Helme R.D. (1996) The impact of dementia on the pain experience. *Pain* **67**, 7–15.

Ferrell B.R. and Ferrell B.A. (eds) (1996) *Pain in the Elderly.* IASP Task Force on Pain in the Elderly. IASP Publications, Seattle.

Gagliese L., Katz J. and Melzack R. (1999) Pain in the elderly. In *The Textbook of Pain* (eds Wall P.D. and Melzack R.). Churchill Livingstone, Edinburgh.

Gibson S.J. and Helme R.D. (1995) Age differences in pain perception and report: a review of physiological, psychological, laboratory and clinical studies. *Pain Reviews* **2**, 111–137.

Jolles J., Verhey F.R., Riedel W.J. and Houx P.J. (1995) Cognitive impairment in elderly people. Predisposing factors and implications for experimental drug studies. *Drugs and Aging* **7**, 459–479.

Macintyre P.E. and Jarvis D.A. (1996) Age is the best predictor of postoperative morphine requirement. *Pain* **64**, 357–364.

Macintyre P.E., Ludbrook G.L. and Upton R. (2000) Acute pain in the elderly. In *Clinical Pain Management: Acute Volume* (eds Rowbotham D. and Macintyre P.). Arnold, London (in press).

Parikh S.S. and Chung F.C. (1995) Postoperative delirium in the elderly. *Anesthesia and Analgesia* **80**, 1223–1231.

Phillips A.C., Polisson R.P. and Simon L.S. (1997) NSAIDs and the elderly: toxicity and economic implications. *Drugs and Aging* **10**, 119–130.

Richardson J. and Bresland K. (1998) The management of postsurgical pain in the elderly population. *Drugs and Aging* **13**, 17–31.

Royal College of Anaesthetists (1998) *Guidelines for the use of non-steroidal anti-inflammatory drugs in the perioperative period.* London: Royal College of Anaesthetists.

CHAPTER 12

EDUCATION

Medical staff

Nursing staff

Patients

One of the well-recognized reasons for past and current deficiencies in the management of acute pain is inadequate education of medical, nursing and allied health staff and students, patients and their families and friends. Inadequate knowledge, misconceptions and the persistence of some of the myths that surround pain management continue to result in barriers that prevent optimal analgesia in many patients (see Chapter 1).

Better education of all groups is needed if more sophisticated methods of pain relief (such as patient-controlled and epidural analgesia) are to be managed safely and effectively and if better results are to be gained from conventional methods of pain relief (such as intermittent opioid injections).

MEDICAL STAFF

Education of junior medical staff should include all aspects of the management of acute pain. While they will not be directly responsible for more advanced, newer methods of pain relief, they must have a sound working knowledge of them. They must be aware of possible complications and drug interactions and be able to explain the techniques to both patients and their relatives. Responsibility for more conventional methods of analgesia is often delegated to junior medical staff. A better understanding of drugs and techniques available will help to improve the effectiveness of these forms of pain relief.

Current teaching usually includes information about anatomy, physiology and theory of pain, but lacks sufficient practical detail.

NURSING STAFF

intro

Ward nurses are directly involved in the management of all forms of pain relief and play a key role in ensuring that analgesia, whether simple or sophisticated, is safely and effectively managed. Education and accreditation programs are therefore essential.

EDUCATION

The education requirements are twofold – general and specialized.

General education

General education will lead to a better practical understanding of drugs and techniques used (including simple techniques). Important topics include early recognition and treatment of side effects, the physiological and psychological benefits of better acute pain management, and the importance of patient education. The appropriate use of nonpharmacological measures should be understood as well as issues arising from the treatment of pain in cognitively impaired patients and in patients from different cultures.

Time available for education within a hospital is often limited. Priorities must therefore be set regarding the importance of various pain topics. It is much more important for nurses to realize that the best measure of pain intensity is the patient's self-report and to understand the principles of opioid titration based on this self-report, than for them to be taught excessive detail about individual drugs or the physiology of pain.

Specialized education

Specialized education leads to safe and effective understanding and management of more sophisticated methods of pain relief such as patient-controlled analgesia (PCA), and epidural or intrathecal analgesia.

ACCREDITATION AND REACCREDITATION

Many institutions require some form of certification or accreditation before registered nurses can assume responsibility for a patient whose pain is being managed using one of the more advanced methods of pain relief listed above.

Accreditation programs usually consist of:
- verbal and written information (e.g. lectures or workshops and booklets)
- written assessment (e.g. multiple choice questionnaires)
- practical assessment (e.g. demonstration of ability to program machines, administer epidural bolus doses)

Reaccreditation every 1–2 years will help ensure that knowledge and practices are regularly updated. Formal education programs need to be supplemented with informal 'one-on-one' teaching in the ward.

PATIENTS

Many patients still rate the fear of pain as their major preoperative concern and many still expect significant pain after surgery. Their attitudes and expectations can affect pain perception and analgesic requirements.

Patients who learn to assess their pain, and are made aware that they should ask for more pain relief when needed, will have more control over the dose and delivery of analgesic drugs, regardless of the analgesic technique used. Appropriate education and information can therefore be a powerful tool in helping to ensure effective pain relief.

Information should be given to each patient and tailored to the needs of that patient. It should include:
- *procedural information*: details of the planned medical or surgical procedure
- *sensory information*: descriptions of the sensory experiences that a patient may expect
- *physiological coping information*: instructions for coping with pain related to activities such as coughing and walking

Adequate education and information can lead to decreases in anxiety, analgesic use and perceptions of pain intensity. For some, however, especially those with high levels of anxiety or poor coping skills (e.g. a tendency to use denial or avoidance to deal with problems), excessive information and the need to make decisions can exacerbate anxiety and pain.

Information can be presented in a number of ways: verbally, in a booklet, or on a video. In general, a mix of these methods probably gives the best results. Although education about pain management should ideally start before it is needed, this will not always be possible (e.g. after an emergency operation or trauma).

It is known that most patients remember only a small part of any information presented at one time. Therefore, it will need to be repeated a number of times, including during treatment.

EDUCATION REQUIREMENTS

The education requirements for patients are twofold – general and specialized.

General education

Patients should be made aware of a number of general factors important to their pain relief. These include the following.

Treatment goals and benefits

Patients should know why effective analgesia is important for their recovery as well as their comfort. The benefits of physiotherapy and early mobilization should be explained. They should be assured that every attempt will be made to make them as comfortable as possible but that pain scores of zero at all times are usually not achievable with medications currently available. Patients should be aware that it is better to treat pain early than to delay treatment until pain is severe.

Options available for the treatment of acute pain

Options available for treatment of acute pain will vary from case to case, but patients should play an active role in expressing their preference after possible risks, benefits and side effects have been explained.

Monitoring pain and its treatment

Methods used in the measurement of pain should be outlined. Patients should know that there is no 'right or wrong' answer for pain scores but that these scores are helpful for tailoring their analgesic requirements. In some patients it may be helpful to explain that excessive sedation means they need a little less opioid.

The need to communicate inadequate analgesia or side effects

Patients should be encouraged to tell their doctors and nurses if analgesia is inadequate or if they are experiencing side effects. If intermittent opioid regimens are being used, the importance of asking for the next dose as soon as they begin to feel uncomfortable should be explained. They should not feel they are 'bothering busy nursing staff'.

Concerns about the risks of addiction

Many patients (or their relatives) are still concerned about the risks of addiction to opioids. Repeated explanations may be required to allay these fears.

Specialized education

Explanations of individual analgesic techniques such as PCA and epidural analgesia should be given, including expected duration of therapy and subsequent analgesic management. The description of PCA does not have to be technically detailed. However, patients must know that they can press the button whenever they are uncomfortable and that they are the only ones allowed to do this (i.e. family and staff are not permitted to do so). Patients should be assured that, despite the use of these techniques, direct personal contact time with nursing staff will not be reduced.

The safety of PCA and 'being in control' must be emphasized. Most of the complications of PCA therapy will be due to the opioids, although an explanation of other causes of some side effects may be useful. For example, a patient experiencing nausea or vomiting after bowel surgery may be reluctant to use PCA if they are told that the only cause of this is the opioid.

The possible side effects and complications of epidural analgesia also should be explained including the need to report to the hospital immediately if increasing back pain or neurological symptoms occur at any time before or after discharge from hospital.

The Agency for Health Care Policy and Research (US Department of Health and Human Services) has issued a booklet titled *Pain Control After Surgery: A Patient's Guide* (Carr *et al.* 1992b). A consumer's guide published by the National Health and Medical Research Council of Australia is also available (websites of both are listed in Appendix 12a).

An example of more specific information given to patients about PCA and epidural analgesia is also included at the end of this chapter.

REFERENCES AND FURTHER READING

Bondy L.R., Sims N., Schroeder D.R. *et al.* (1999) The effect of anesthetic patient education in preoperative patient anxiety. *Regional Anesthesia and Pain Medicine* **24**, 158–164.

Carr D.B., Jacox A.K., Chapman C.R. et al. (1992a) *Acute Pain Management: Operative or Medical Procedures and Trauma, Clinical Practice Guideline.* AHCPR Pub. No. 92–0032. Rockville, MD: Agency for Health Care Policy and Research, Public Health Service, US Department of Health and Human Services.

Carr D.B., Jacox A.K., Chapman C.R. et al. (1992b) Acute Pain Management Guideline Panel. *Pain Control After Surgery: A Patient's Guide.* AHCPR Pub. No. 92–0021. Rockville, MD: Agency for Health Care Policy and Research, Public Health Service, US Department of Health and Human Services.

Ferrell B.R. (1996) Patient education and non-drug interventions. In *Pain in the Elderly* (eds Ferrell B.R. and Ferrell B.A.). IASP Task Force on Pain in the Elderly. IASP Publications, Seattle.

McCaffery M. and Ferrell B.R. (1997) Nurses' knowledge of pain assessment and management: how much progress have we made? *Journal of Pain and Symptom Management* **14**, 175–188.

National Health and Medical Research Council (1999) *Acute Pain Management: The Scientific Evidence.* Canberra (available at http://www.nhmrc.health.gov.au/publicat/pdf/cp57.pdf).

National Health and Medical Research Council (1999) *Acute Pain Management: Information for Consumers.* Canberra (available at http://www.nhmrc.health.gov.au/publicat/pdf/cp58.pdf).

Warfield C.A. and Kahn C.H. (1995) Acute pain management programs in US hospitals and experiences and attitudes among US adults. *Anesthesiology* **83**, 1090–1094.

APPENDIX TO CHAPTER 12

Examples of patient and staff educational material.

12A Examples of consumer information available on the internet

12B *Patient-Controlled Analgesia (PCA) and Epidural Analgesia* – a patient information sheet published by the Royal Adelaide Hospital Acute Pain Service

12C Self-assessment questions suitable for use as part of an accreditation program

APPENDIX 12A

Examples of consumer information available on the internet

1. National Health and Medical Research Council of Australia
   'Acute Pain Management: Information for Consumers'
   http://www.nhmrc.health.gov.au/publicat/pdf/cp58.pdf

2. Agency for Health Care Policy and Research, US
   Department of Health and Human Services
   'Pain Control after Surgery: an Patient's Guide' (AHCPR
   Pub. No. 92–0021)
   http://text.nlm.nib.gov
   select 'AHCPR Supported Guidelines' to find 'Acute Pain
   Management: Consumers Guide'

1/1/93

Acute Pain Service
Royal Adelaide Hospital

PATIENT INFORMATION

PATIENT-CONTROLLED ANALGESIA (PCA) AND EPIDURAL ANALGESIA

The management of acute pain, particularly pain following more major operations or accidents, has improved quite significantly over the past few years. No longer are injections into your arm or leg the only way of giving strong pain killing drugs.

You may be offered one of these new pain relieving methods to help treat your pain. Here at the Royal Adelaide Hospital the two most commonly used of these methods are **patient-controlled analgesia** (called PCA for short) and **epidural analgesia.**

Analgesia means "painlessness" or "no pain". Unfortunately, with the drugs that are currently available, it is usually *not* possible to safely relieve *all* the pain. Instead, we aim for enough pain relief to make you *comfortable*, so that you can sleep, move around and, very importantly, do coughing and deep breathing and other physiotherapy exercises.

The **Acute Pain Service (APS)** is part of the Department of Anaesthesia at the Royal Adelaide Hospital. Anaesthetists are the doctors who look after your anaesthetic during your operation, but they also specialise in pain relief. If you have one of the newer forms of pain relief you will be seen at least once a day by an anaesthetist and nurse from the APS in addition the doctors and nurses who provide your regular ward care. The APS also has an anaesthetist on-call 24 hours a day.

Is pain relief important?
Yes. As well as making patients more comfortable, good pain relief can help speed recovery. This is especially true for patients having more major operations.

APPENDIX 12B

PATIENT-CONTROLLED ANALGESIA (PCA)

PCA means that you actually have control over your own pain relief. There is a machine called a PCA pump that can be used to give a small dose of a strong pain killer, such as morphine or pethidine. Usually this machine will be attached to the drip (intravenous line) in your arm. If you are uncomfortable you press a button and the machine will pump a small dose of the drug into this line. You can do this whenever you are uncomfortable - you do not need to tell the nurse first. The amount of drug delivered by the machine each time you press the button, as well as other settings on the machine, will be ordered by the anaesthetist from the Acute Pain Service. The PCA machine will be programmed by your nurse according to these orders.

How often can I press the button?
You can press the PCA button whenever you feel uncomfortable. However, once the button has been pushed and the PCA machine has delivered the dose (this takes about 1 minute) the machine will "lockout" for 5 minutes. This means that, even if you push the button within this "lockout" time of 5 minutes, the PCA machine will not respond. This is so that you have time to feel the effect of one dose of pain relieving drug before getting another dose. Remember, the aim is to make yourself comfortable - it is not always possible to be completely pain free.

Who is allowed to press the PCA button?
The patient is the ONLY person allowed to press the button. Do not allow ANY hospital staff, relatives or friends to do so.

Will the pain relieving drug work immediately?
No. These drugs need to get to the brain and spinal cord and it may take 5 minutes or longer for the drug to work fully. However, this is still much quicker than if these drugs were given by injection into your arm or leg. If you are about to do something that you know will hurt, like coughing or moving, press the PCA button about 5 minutes *before* doing it.

What if the pain relieving drug doesn't work?
If you are pressing the PCA button quite frequently and are still uncomfortable tell your nurse, who will firstly check that the drip is running properly. As long as you are not sleepy your nurse can increase the

APPENDIX 12B

amount of drug you get when you press the button. If necessary, the Acute Pain Service will be consulted.

Can I overdose?

PCA is probably one of the safest ways of giving strong pain killing drugs. The dose of drug that you get with each press of the button is very small so if you were getting just a little too much you would feel sleepy. This means that you would not press the button again. Your nurse would also notice this and would reduce the amount of drug delivered with each push of the button and, if necessary, treat the sleepiness. The amount of pain relieving drug that is needed varies greatly between patients so it is not unusual to have to make alterations in the dose.

Can I get addicted?

When drugs like morphine and pethidine are used to treat acute pain like the pain after operations or accidents, the risk of addiction is negligible. It is very important *not* to let the fear of addiction stop you from using enough of the drugs to be comfortable or to stop you from moving or coughing.

Will I feel nauseated or vomit?

There are many reasons for feeling sick after operations - drugs like morphine and pethidine are only one possible cause. Whatever the cause, you will be ordered other drugs called *antiemetics* that can help counteract the nausea or vomiting. If one of these drugs doesn't work your nurse will try another. If the morphine or pethidine does seem to be causing the problem, or at least making it worse, it is often because the dose of the drug is a little high. There doesn't seem to be a great difference between these two drugs and for this reason we will often decrease the dose that you get from each press of the PCA button, or increase the time the PCA machine takes to deliver the drug. Occasionally, it may help to change the drug.

For how long will I use PCA?

Normally PCA will continue while you have your drip in. When your doctors on the ward allow you to drink it means that the drip may soon be removed. PCA will usually stop at this time but you will be ordered other pain relieving drugs should you need them. Commonly these pain killers will be tablets. The type and number of tablets will depend of how much pain relieving drug you used with PCA.

APPENDIX 12B

EPIDURAL ANALGESIA

You may already know about epidural analgesia as it is a method often used to treat pain during childbirth. This same technique can also be used to treat pain after some operations and accidents. Most pain relieving drugs work by acting on the brain and spinal cord and they are carried there in the blood stream. With an epidural, the use of a very small plastic tube means that these drugs can be placed close to the spinal cord and nerves so that the drugs can act directly on them and not have to travel to them in the blood stream. This method of pain relief is one of the best available but it is not necessary after all operations or accidents. If you have an epidural for pain relief it will be put in by your anaesthetist, who will explain the procedure to you beforehand.

What pain relieving drugs are used with an epidural?
Two types of drugs are used - drugs like morphine and pethidine or drugs called local anaesthetics. Most often we use a mixture of the two types of drugs.

What if the epidural doesn't work?
If you are uncomfortable tell your nurse who will check the epidural and can increase the amount of drug that you are getting. If necessary, the Acute Pain Service may also be contacted.

Will my legs feel numb, weak or heavy?
If you are having an operation, the epidural will often be used as part of the anaesthetic as well as for pain relief afterwards. A strong local anaesthetic drug may be given during the operation so immediately after the operation your legs may feel numb and heavy. This will wear off in a few hours. The drugs that we use for pain relief in an epidural after the operation will not be as strong so your legs should feel virtually normal. If they do not, let your nurse know. The aim is to keep you comfortable but still able to move around in bed, sit out of bed and even walk, if your doctors allow it.

Will my legs be numb, weak or heavy when I leave hospital?
NO. In the unlikely event that you have gone home and notice persistent tingling, numbness, heaviness or weakness in your legs, or have trouble passing water, or have a pain in your back that is getting worse, you should tell your doctor immediately and ask him/her to contact the APS at the Royal Adelaide Hospital.

SELF-ASSESSMENT

As noted in Chapter 12, nursing education and accreditation programs are important if acute pain is to be managed safely and effectively. In particular, such programs are recommended if techniques such as patient-controlled and epidural analgesia are to be made available on general hospital wards. The questions below are examples of ones that might be used as part of an accreditation assessment.

Select the *one best answer* from the four options listed for each question.

1. Potential adverse effects of pain after surgery include:
   a. decreased myocardial oxygen consumption
   b. hypoxemia
   c. hypotension
   d. sedation

2. Unreliable measures of pain include:
   a. observation of patient behaviour
   b. the verbal numerical rating scale
   c. the categorical rating scale
   d. the visual analog scale

3. Effects of opioid receptor activation include:
   a. physical dependence, mediated via the mu receptor
   b. pruritus, mediated via the kappa receptor
   c. respiratory depression, mediated via the delta receptor
   d. nausea and vomiting, mediated via the kappa receptor

4. A dose of IM codeine that gives a similar degree of pain relief as 10 mg IM morphine is:
   a. 10 mg
   b. 60 mg
   c. 130 mg
   d. 200 mg

5. A dose of oral codeine that gives a similar degree of pain relief as 10 mg IM morphine is:
   a. 10 mg
   b. 60 mg
   c. 130 mg
   d. 200 mg

6. A dose of oral morphine that gives a similar degree of pain relief as 10 mg IM morphine is:
   a. 3 mg
   b. 10 mg
   c. 30 mg
   d. 100 mg

7. The best early clinical indicator of opioid-induced respiratory depression is:
   a. increasing sedation
   b. confusion
   c. upper airway obstruction
   d. a decrease in respiratory rate

8. Causes of hypoxemia in the postoperative period include:
   a. opioid-related obstructive apnea
   b. postoperative changes in lung function
   c. rebound REM sleep
   d. all of the above

9. A patient wakes easily when you go to give him his medications but he appears drowsy and keeps falling asleep while you are talking to him. His sedation score is:

a. 0
b. 1
c. 2
d. 3

10. A patient is wide awake and has been watching television all afternoon. His sedation score is:

a. 0
b. 1
c. 2
d. 3

11. The best predictor of the amount of morphine a patient is likely to need after major surgery is:

a. gender of the patient
b. age of the patient
c. weight of the patient
d. estimated lean body weight of the patient

12. In a population of 20-year-old patients undergoing major surgery, the expected average 24-hour morphine requirement in the first day after surgery is:

a. 15 mg
b. 30 mg
c. 60 mg
d. 80 mg

13. In a population of 70-year-old patients undergoing major surgery, the expected average 24-hour morphine requirement in the first day after surgery is:

a. 15 mg
b. 30 mg
c. 60 mg
d. 80 mg

14. If an injection of morphine is given IV, the average time for the full effect of the morphine to be seen is:
    a. 30 seconds
    b. 1 minute
    c. 5 minutes
    d. 15 minutes

15. If an injection of fentanyl is given IV, the average time for the full effect of the fentanyl to be seen is:
    a. 30 seconds
    b. 1 minute
    c. 5 minutes
    d. 15 minutes

16. Morphine 6-glucuronide (M6G) is a metabolite of morphine. M6G:
    a. has no analgesic activity
    b. does not accumulate in renal failure
    c. has the same spectrum of side effects as morphine
    d. has a shorter half-life than morphine

17. Codeine is a naturally occurring alkaloid of opium. Codeine:
    a. will not result in effective analgesia in 50% of white patients
    b. has a high affinity for the opioid receptor
    c. is useful for the treatment of severe pain
    d. is metabolized in the liver where 10% is converted to morphine

18. Normeperidine (norpethidine) is a metabolite of meperidine. Early signs and symptoms of normeperidine toxicity:
    a. include sedation
    b. include agitation
    c. are reversible using naloxone
    d. result from activation of opioid receptors

19. Agonist-antagonist opioid drugs:
    a. can precipitate a withdrawal syndrome in patients on long-term opioid agonist therapy
    b. cause less sedation than opioid agonist drugs
    c. include propoxyphene
    d. include buprenorphine

20. When morphine is given by intermittent SC injection:
    a. absorption into the blood stream will be slower than following an IM morphine injection
    b. higher doses of morphine will be needed than if given by IM injection
    c. morphine should be given in the smallest volume possible
    d. repeat injections must not be given for another 4 hours

21. A 23-year-old patient is prescribed '7.5–15 mg SC morphine 2-hourly PRN' for pain relief after a laparotomy for a ruptured spleen the day before. He is wide awake and watching television. His last injection of morphine was 12.5 mg 2 hours ago. He says his pain score is 9 and that he would like another injection of the same dose of morphine. You would:
    a. suggest he wait another hour
    b. give 15 mg morphine
    c. give 7.5 mg morphine
    d. give 12.5 mg morphine

22. A patient who is wide awake complains of pain 10 minutes after an IM injection of morphine and asks for another injection. You:
    a. tell him you will give him another injection now
    b. tell him that the injection has not yet had a chance to work
    c. tell him he must wait another 2 hours
    d. tell him he must wait another 3 hours

23. A patient is ordered 10 mg IM morphine 'strictly 4-hourly'. When the patient is due her next injection it is noted that she has a sedation score of 2. You decide the best course of action is to:

    a. give the injection as ordered
    b. give 5 mg morphine only
    c. give naloxone
    d. withhold the injection

24. An 80-year-old patient is given an IM injection of 10 mg morphine. One hour later she is noted to have a sedation score of 3. You are asked to give naloxone. An appropriate dose and route would be:

    a. 100 µg naloxone IM
    b. 100 µg naloxone IV
    c. 400 µg naloxone IV
    d. 100 mg naloxone IV

25. A continuous infusion of morphine is ordered at a rate of 2 mg/h. On average, the full effect of morphine given at that rate of infusion will be seen within:

    a. 15 minutes
    b. 1 hour
    c. 4 hours
    d. 15 hours

26. Transdermal fentanyl patches enable fentanyl to be absorbed through the skin. These patches:

    a. have an effect that may last 24 hours after the patch is removed
    b. allow blood concentrations of fentanyl to rise rapidly
    c. are useful in the routine management of acute pain
    d. have only small amounts of fentanyl left in the patch after removal

27. Controlled-release tablets of oral morphine:
   a. take 3 hours or more to reach peak blood levels after administration
   b. are ordered '4-hourly PRN'
   c. are suitable for the rapid titration of pain relief
   d. are more potent than morphine syrup (i.e. a smaller dose is needed to give the same analgesic effect)

28. A patient using PCA with a bolus dose of 2 mg morphine (lock-out 6 minutes) complains of repeatedly waking in severe pain at night. He is receiving, on average, 8 mg every hour (i.e. four 'successful' demands). You would:
   a. tell him to press the demand button more frequently, as he can get more doses from the machine each hour
   b. suspect he has an addiction to morphine
   c. tell him that an increase in the size of the bolus dose is not appropriate
   d. consider the use of a continuous (background) infusion

29. A patient using PCA with a bolus dose of 2 mg morphine (lock-out 6 minutes) complains of severe pain. He is receiving, on average, 8 mg every hour (i.e. four 'successful' demands). He has a sedation score of 2. You would:
   a. tell him to press the demand button more frequently, as he can get more doses from the machine each hour
   b. decrease the size of the bolus dose
   c. increase the lock-out interval
   d. consider the use of a continuous (background) infusion

30. A patient using PCA with a bolus dose of 2 mg morphine (lock-out 6 minutes) complains of severe nausea and vomiting a few minutes after he presses the demand button. He is receiving, on average, 2 mg every hour (i.e. one 'successful' demand). You would:
    a. tell him to press the demand button less frequently
    b. decrease the size of the bolus dose
    c. increase the lock-out interval
    d. stop PCA and give morphine by intermittent SC injection

31. A patient using PCA morphine complains of severe itching over his face and chest. A decision is made to change to PCA fentanyl. If the bolus dose of morphine is currently 1 mg, an appropriate bolus dose of fentanyl would be:
    a. 1 µg
    b. 5 µg
    c. 20 µg
    d. 50 µg

32. A decision is made to change a patient from PCA morphine to PCA tramadol. If the bolus dose of morphine is currently 1 mg, an appropriate bolus dose of tramadol would be:
    a. 1 mg
    b. 5 mg
    c. 10 mg
    d. 20 mg

33. A patient using PCA morphine is tolerating oral fluids and the decision is made to change to oral oxycodone. The patient has used 75 mg PCA morphine in the preceding 24 hours. An appropriate order for oral oxycodone would be:
    a. 5–10 mg 4-hourly PRN
    b. 5–25 mg 4-hourly PRN
    c. 5–25 mg 6-hourly PRN
    d. 5–10 mg 6-hourly PRN

34. A patient using PCA morphine is tolerating oral fluids and the decision is made to change to morphine syrup. The patient has used 75 mg PCA morphine in the preceding 24 hours. The equivalent of this dose in morphine syrup would be:

    a. 25 mg in 24 hours
    b. 75 mg in 24 hours
    c. 150 mg in 24 hours
    d. 225 mg in 24 hours

35. A dose of epidural morphine that gives a similar degree of pain relief as 5 mg IM morphine is:

    a. 0.1 mg
    b. 0.5 mg
    c. 1 mg
    d. 5 mg

36. A dose of intrathecal morphine that gives a similar degree of pain relief as 5 mg IM morphine is:

    a. 0.1 mg
    b. 0.5 mg
    c. 1 mg
    d. 5 mg

37. Epidural opioids cause:

    a. less nausea and vomiting than epidural local anesthetics
    b. more itching than epidural local anesthetics
    c. more hypotension than epidural local anesthetics
    d. less sedation than epidural local anesthetics

38. Postdural puncture headache is typically:

    a. bifrontal or occipital
    b. usually worse when lying down, compared with sitting
    c. a result of leakage of blood into the epidural space
    d. more likely in older patients

39. A patient is receiving an epidural infusion of bupivacaine 0.1% and fentanyl 5 μg/ml at a rate of 10 ml/h for postoperative analgesia. His operation was 2 days ago. He tells you that he has some numbness in his left leg. You would:
   a. tell him that it is likely to be due to the bupivacaine
   b. cease the infusion or reduce the rate of infusion
   c. consider the possibility of epidural hematoma or epidural abscess
   d. all of the above

40. A patient is receiving an epidural infusion of bupivacaine 0.1% and fentanyl 5 μg/ml at a rate of 10 ml/h for postoperative analgesia. His operation was 2 days ago. You note that his blood pressure is 80 mmHg systolic (it had been 130). You would:
   a. tell him that it is likely to be due to the bupivacaine
   b. administer naloxone
   c. consider the possibility of postoperative bleeding
   d. all of the above

41. A patient calls you from her home at 10 p.m. She has increasing back pain and is having trouble voiding. She says that she had an epidural anesthetic for her hysterectomy 5 weeks ago. You would:
   a. tell her to come to your hospital first thing tomorrow morning
   b. tell her that back pain is a common problem after epidural anesthesia and that she should take two acetaminophen (paracetamol) tablets every 4 hours
   c. tell her that she must come into the hospital immediately for an MRI scan
   d. tell her that she must come into the hospital immediately for some antibiotics

42. Nonsteroidal anti-inflammatory drugs (NSAIDs) inhibit the enyzme cyclo-oxygenase (COX). There are two types of COX, COX-1 and COX-2:
   a. COX-1 is produced as a result of tissue injury or inflammation
   b. COX-1 is responsible for the adverse effects of NSAIDs on renal function
   c. COX-2 is responsible for the adverse effects of NSAIDs on platelet function
   d. COX-2 is constitutive

43. Risk factors for the development of renal failure in association with the use of NSAIDs include:
   a. hypotension
   b. low urine output
   c. cardiac failure
   d. all of the above

44. Risk factors for the development of gastric erosions following the use of NSAIDs include:
   a. concurrent use of misoprostol
   b. history of peptic ulcer disease
   c. the use of the oral rather the rectal or intravenous routes for administration of the drugs
   d. all of the above

45. Acetaminophen (paracetamol):
   a. should be used with caution in patients with chronic alcoholism
   b. is recommended for administration in doses up to 8 g/day
   c. has analgesic, antipyretic and anti-inflammatory activity
   d. is more effective when given by the rectal than the oral route

46. Ketamine:
    a. acts on NMDA and opioid receptors
    b. is ineffective in the treatment of neuropathic pain
    c. increases tolerance to opioids
    d. has a high incidence of central nervous system side effects when used in low doses (e.g. 100 mg/day)

47. Nitrous oxide is sometimes used as analgesia for short painful procedures. Contraindications to the use of nitrous oxide include:
    a. concurrent use of opioids
    b. vitamin C deficiency
    c. pneumothorax
    d. iron-deficiency anemia

48. A patient has become physically dependent on opioids. This means that:
    a. they will suffer withdrawal signs and symptoms if naloxone is given
    b. they will need progressively larger doses of opioid to get the same effect
    c. they will seek drugs from nonmedical sources
    d. they take the drugs to experience a 'high'

49. A patient is admitted following a motorbike accident. He has no movement in his right arm and an injury to his brachial plexus is suspected. Four days later he says that he has burning and shooting pains in his arm. He also says that the morphine he is getting is not helping the pain nearly as much as it was before. This type of pain is called:
    a. nociceptive pain
    b. neuropathic pain
    c. psychological pain
    d. phantom pain

50. Drugs that are used in the treatment of phantom pain include:
   a. amitriptyline
   b. ketamine
   c. carbamazepine
   d. all of the above

Answers

1.	b	14.	d	27.	a	40.	c
2.	a	15.	c	28.	d	41.	c
3.	a	16.	c	29.	b	42.	b
4.	c	17.	d	30.	b	43.	d
5.	d	18.	b	31.	c	44.	b
6.	c	19.	a	32.	c	45.	a
7.	a	20.	c	33.	b	46.	a
8.	d	21.	d	34.	d	47.	c
9.	c	22.	b	35.	c	48.	a
10.	a	23.	d	36.	a	49.	b
11.	b	24.	b	37.	b	50.	d
12.	d	25.	d	38.	a		
13.	b	26.	a	39.	d		